TOTAL REVISION FOR THE PRIMARY FRCA

2nd Edition

Yogen Amin
Roger Cordery
Mike Davies
Annie Hunningher
Tim Isitt

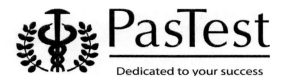

PasTest

Dedicated to your success

© 2008 PASTEST LTD

Egerton Court
Parkgate Estate
Knutsford
Cheshire
WA16 8DX
Telephone: 01565 752000

A percentage of the questions were previously published in *FRCA Primary Practice Papers*.

First published 2008

ISBN: 1904627943
      978 1904627994

A catalogue record for this book is available from the British Library.

The information contained within this book was obtained by the author from reliable sources. However, while every effort has been made to ensure its accuracy, no responsibility for loss, damage or injury occasioned to any person acting or refraining from action as a result of information contained herein can be accepted by the publishers or author.

PasTest Revision Books and Intensive Courses

PasTest has been established in the field of postgraduate medical education since 1972, providing revision books and intensive study courses for doctors preparing for their professional examinations.

Books and courses are available for the following specialties:
MRCGP, MRCP Parts 1 and 2, MRCPCH Parts 1 and 2, MRCS, MRCOG Parts 1 and 2, DRCOG, DCH, FRCA, PLAB Parts 1 and 2, Dentistry.

For further details contact:
PasTest, Freepost, Knutsford, Cheshire WA16 7BR
Tel: 01565 752000   Fax: 01565 650264
www.pastest.co.uk   enquiries@pastest.co.uk

Text prepared by Saxon Graphics Ltd, Derby
Printed and bound in the UK by CPI Antony Rowe

7 day loan

This book is due for return on or before the last date shown below.

Dedication

We would like to thank our friends and family for their support in putting together this book.

We would also like to dedicate this book to those intrepid exam-takers. We've been there and we know how challenging it can be, but also how rewarding. We hope this book will arm you with confidence for the exams and you'll pass with flying colours!

Yogen Amin
Roger Cordery
Mike Davies
Annie Hunningher

Contents

Contents

About the Authors

Yogen Amin BSc, MB ChB, FRCA is a Consultant Neuroanaesthetist and Neurointensivist at The National Hospital for Neurology and Neurosurgery, and Honorary Senior Lecturer at University College London and The Institute of Neurology, Queen Square. After 3 years pre-clinical at St Andrews University he graduated from Manchester University in 1993. He trained as an Anaesthetist at the Imperial School of Anaesthesia, during this period he was involved in research at The Magill Department of Anaesthesia, Imperial College, London and at Stanford University, Palo Alto, California.

Roger Cordery AKC, MB BS (Lond), FRCA qualified from King's College School of Medicine and Dentistry in 1994. He is now a Consultant Anaesthetist and Honorary Senior Lecturer at University College London and the Heart Hospitals. His main interests include regional anaesthesia and analgesia, perioperative transoesophageal echocardiography, transfusion medicine and medical education at both undergraduate and postgraduate levels. He is never knowingly underdressed!

Mike Davies MB BS (Lond), BSc (UCL), FRCA is currently working as a specialist registrar in anaesthetics at the Heart Hospital in London, having finished a year at University College Hospital as an education fellow. He is at present doing an MA in clinical education at the Institute of Education, London.

Annie Hunningher MB ChB, FRCA, trained at the University of Manchester and is doing her postgraduate training in London, currently as a year 5 SpR in Anaesthesia. Her areas of special interest include teaching and difficult airways.

Tim Isitt MRCP, FRCA, is a Consultant Anaesthetist at the Luton and Dunstable Hospital, and The Portland Hospital for Women and Children, London. He is an Honorary Senior Lecturer at University College, London. His main interests are Obstetric Anaesthesia, Undergraduate and Postgraduate education.

We are always grateful for notification of any mistakes or discrepancies that appear in our books. If you do find an item which you suspect may be incorrect please notify the Publisher in writing so that we can ensure that any mistake is rectified when the book is reprinted.

INTRODUCTION

This revised and updated version of Tim Isitt's book aims to reflect changes in anaesthesia and in the Primary FRCA examination.

The exam requires dedication and commitment to pass. The best way to do this is to have a thorough understanding and knowledge of all parts of the syllabus.

This book aims to allow you, 'the candidate', to practise techniques and consolidate your knowledge. It can also be a useful book in a study group where you can practise answering questions and being the examiner, which gives you valuable insight into how to present your answers. You can annotate the book to make topics clearer for you to understand and remember. You can also invent related questions that follow the same approach. For example 'What are the properties of the ideal induction agent?' can also be related to neuromuscular blockers and other commonly used groups of drugs. This will help you to remember a structure around which to base your answer. Classification and a methodical presentation of your answer is a skill that requires practise. The need for practise (especially as the exam approaches) as well as revision cannot be overemphasised. It is important to seize any opportunity you can to ask colleagues to question you and to attend practice courses.

When to sit the exam
Candidates need 12 months of approved training in the United Kingdom or Republic of Ireland before they can sit the Primary FRCA examination. It is generally recommended to complete 18 months of training prior to sitting the exam. Candidates may not sit the Primary FRCA examination more than four times. Those who fail the exam twice are referred for advice from the college. Further information can be obtained at http://www.rcoa.ac.uk/

THE EXAMINATION
MCQs (Multiple Choice Questions)
There are some changes that will occur to the Examinations Regulations over the next 3 years, so it would be worth keeping up to date with these in the Examinations section at the Royal College website, http://www.rcoa.ac.uk.

Each paper has 90 questions, each with 5 stems, to be completed in 3 hours:

30 in Physiology and Biochemistry
30 in Pharmacology
30 in Physics and Clinical Measurement.

By practising these papers you can find the MCQ technique that suits you best. The paper is negatively marked so it is hazardous to guess. NB. From September 2008 the negative marking will be removed. 'The don't know' option will be removed, you will only be offered a 'T' of 'F' option for each question. Marks will NOT be deducted for wrong answers.

OSCEs (Objective Structured Clinical Examinations)
The number of OSCEs has changed from 16 to 18. At the time of the exam only 16 stations are live but the examiners don't know which stations are being marked and which are not.

Most questions in the OSCEs are factually based and therefore quite straight-forward, even if the whole procedure is quite intense. They cover a wide range of topics including data interpretation, anatomy, clinical exami-nation, history taking, equipment etc.

The simulation station, the 'Sim man', is a new addition and is used to test routine evaluation of physical signs as well as emergency situations and critical incidents.

The communication station is designed to test just that. However, there is a tendency to get bogged down in the medical details which prevent you scoring points. The examiners will try, where they are able, to redirect you if you are going wildly off track, but you should learn to recognise the difference between history taking stations and communication stations and ensure that you answer them appropriately.

SOEs (Structured Oral Examinations)
The SOEs are in two parts SOE1 and SOE2, each lasting 30 minutes.

Remember to speak clearly and classify, classify, classify!

As well as questioning you the examiner may show you pictures or ask you to draw relevant diagrams during the exam. Draw big! It is worth practising drawings and remembering to always label the axis first when drawing graphs. It is also important to learn definitions and laws that the examiner may ask you to recite. Try not to launch into a related topic that you don't know much about as you could find yourself struggling. Always try to start an answer with a classification or brief overview as this also gives you time to order your answer. It is important to look interested in the subject matter and bring it to life! Don't fiddle or look down as it will put you off as well as the examiner. Watch out for top tips in boxes in the suggested answers.

SOE1

This part of the exam consists of four questions in physiology followed by four questions in pharmacology. The first examiner asks questions whilst the second examiner takes notes and they then swap roles for the second part of the SOE1. Three topics will be covered in each half of the SOE making a total of six topics in this part of the exam.

SOE2

This part of the exam consists of four questions in physics and clinical measurement followed by questions in clinical anaesthesia, including a structured clinical case study with a critical incident. (You will be given a copy of the scenario to read 5 minutes before entering the examination.)

List of critical incident and anaesthetic emergencies

The book also includes a list of possible critical incidents and anaesthetic emergencies which it is well worth working through on your own so you are ready for anything in the exam as well as your working life!

The primary exam topics are also beloved subjects in the final exam and so a good level of knowledge will provide you with an excellent grounding in your anaesthetic training.

Confidence plays a big part in the exam and the best way to achieve it is by thorough preparation and perseverance.

'Self-confidence is the first requisite to great undertakings.'
Samuel Johnson *(1709-1784) British author.*

You can do it!

Yogen Amin
Roger Cordery
Mike Davies
Annie Hunningher

Abbreviations

5-HT	5-Hydroxytryptamine (Serotonin)
AAGBI	Association of Anaesthetists of Great Britain and Ireland
ABG	arterial blood gas
ACh	acetylcholine
ACT	activated clotting time
ACTH	adrenocorticotrophic hormone
ADH	antidiuretic hormone
ADR	adverse drug reaction
AF	atrial fibrillation
ALI	acute lung injury
aPTT	activated partial thromboplastin time
ARDS	acute respiratory distress syndrome
BE	base excess
BMR	basal metabolic rate
BP	blood pressure
CAPD	citrate, adenine, phosphate and dextrose
CC	closing capacity
CMV	cytomegalovirus
CN	cranial nerve
CO	cardiac output
COP	colloid oncotic pressure
COPD	chronic obstructive pulmonary disease
CPD	citrate, phosphate and dextrose
CPR	cardiopulmonary resuscitation
CSF	cerebrospinal fluid
CSL	compound sodium lactate
CTZ	Chemoreceptor Trigger Zone
CVP	central venous pressure
CXR	chest radiograph
DGH	District General Hospital
DIC	disseminated intravascular coagulation
DOB	date of birth
2,3-DPG	2,3-diphosphoglycerate
DPPC	dipalmitoyl phosphatidyl choline
DVT	deep vein thrombosis
EDP	End Diastolic Point
EDPVR	End Diastolic Pressure-Volume Relationship

Abbreviations

EDV	End Diastolic Volume
EMLA	Eutectic Mixture of Local Anaesthetics
EPs	evoked potentials
ERV	expiratory reserve volume
ESP	End Systolic Point
ESPVR	End Systolic Pressure-Volume Relationship
ESV	End Systolic Volume
ETT	endotracheal tube
FBC	full blood count
FEV_1	forced expiratory volume in 1 second
FFA	free fatty acids
FFP	fresh frozen plasma
FGF	fresh gas flow
FRC	functional residual capacity
FVC	forced vital capacity
G6PD	glucose 6-phosphate dehydrogenase
GA	general anaesthetic
GCS	Glasgow Coma Score
GFR	glomerular filtration rate
HME	heat moisture exchanger
5-HT	5-hydroxytryptamine
IABP	intra-aortic balloon pump
IC	inspiratory capacity
ICP	intracranial pressure
INR	international normalised ratio
IPPV	intermittent positive-pressure ventilation
ITU	intensive therapy unit
IVRA	intravenous regional anaesthesia
JVP	Jugular Venous Pulse
LMA	laryngeal mask airway
LV	left ventricle
MAC	minimum alveolar concentration
MH	malignant hyperthermia
MUA	manipulation under anaesthetic
NA	Noradrenaline
NBM	nil by mouth
NG	nasogastric
NIBP	non-invasive blood pressure
NMDA	N-methyl-D-aspartate
NSAID	non-steroidal anti-inflammatory drug
ODP	operating department practitioner

Abbreviations

PAH	*para*-aminohippuric acid
PAP	pulmonary artery pressure
PCWP	pulmonary capillary wedge pressure
PDPH	post-dural puncture headache
PEEP	positive end-expiratory pressure
PEFR	peak expiratory flow rate
PET	Pre-Eclamptic Toxemia
PICU	paediatric ITU
PONV	postoperative nausea and vomiting
PT	prothrombin time
PTT	partial thromboplastin time
RA	regional anaesthesia
RER	respiratory exchange ratio
RQ	respiratory quotient
RTI	respiratory tract infection
RV	residual volume
Rx	treatment
SAGM	saline, adenine, glucose and mannitol
SNP	sodium nitroprusside
SV	stroke volume
SVC	superior vena cava
SVP	saturated vapour pressure
SVR	systemic vascular resistance
SVT	supraventricular tachycardia
TEG	thromboelastograph
TENS	transcutaneous nerve stimulation
TLC	total lung capacity
TOE	transoesophageal echo
TPN	total parenteral nutrition
TPR	total peripheral resistance
TSH	thyroid stimulating hormone
TT	thrombin time
TURP	transurethral resection of the prostate
TV	Tidal volume
U&Es	urea and electrolytes
VC	Vital Capacity
VIC	vaporiser inside the circle
VOC	vaporiser outside the circle

Multiple Choice Question Paper 1

90 Questions: time allowed 3 hours.

Indicate your answers with a tick or cross in the spaces provided.

1.1 Dopamine antagonists

- ❏ A increase gastric emptying
- ❏ B cause tachyarrhythmias
- ❏ C cause extrapyramidal effects
- ❏ D cause renal artery dilation
- ❏ E are anti-emetic

1.2 Diamorphine

- ❏ A is less potent than morphine
- ❏ B is not used in terminal illness because it is addictive
- ❏ C is more rapid in action than morphine
- ❏ D is more euphoric than morphine
- ❏ E has a high first-pass metabolism

1.3 Alfentanil

- ❏ A is more potent than fentanyl
- ❏ B is more lipid soluble than fentanyl
- ❏ C causes myocardial depression
- ❏ D may cause muscle rigidity
- ❏ E is more rapid in action than fentanyl

1.4 Methohexitone

- ❏ A is a thiobarbiturate
- ❏ B is contraindicated in acute intermittent porphyria
- ❏ C is less potent than thiopentone
- ❏ D is protein bound
- ❏ E is excreted unchanged in the urine

1.5 Propofol

- [ ] A is presented in 10% soya bean oil
- [ ] B decreases blood pressure mainly by vasodilatation
- [ ] C is broken down by plasma cholinesterase
- [ ] D has a standard induction dose of 4–5 mg/kg in healthy adults
- [ ] E is more respiratory depressant than thiopentone

1.6 Regarding non-depolarising neuromuscular block

- [ ] A fasciculation occurs prior to blockade
- [ ] B neostigmine acts by inhibiting the breakdown of acetylcholine
- [ ] C partial block is indicated by post-tetanic facilitation
- [ ] D metabolic acidosis may cause prolongation
- [ ] E aminoglycoside antibiotics cause prolongation

1.7 Atracurium

- [ ] A is metabolised by ester hydrolysis
- [ ] B metabolism is slowed by hypothermia
- [ ] C breakdown produces laudanosine
- [ ] D in larger doses is faster in onset than suxamethonium
- [ ] E at a decreased pH has increased shelf life

1.8 Positive inotropic agents include

- [ ] A glucagon
- [ ] B potassium
- [ ] C verapamil
- [ ] D propranolol
- [ ] E theophylline

1.9 The following are metabolised in the liver

- [ ] A morphine
- [ ] B atracurium
- [ ] C procaine
- [ ] D thiopentone
- [ ] E vecuronium

1.10 Bupivacaine

- ❏ A is more potent than lignocaine
- ❏ B has a longer duration of action than lignocaine
- ❏ C is contraindicated in intravenous regional anaesthesia
- ❏ D is highly protein bound
- ❏ E cardiotoxicity is associated with the D stereoisomer

1.11 Enzyme induction occurs with

- ❏ A phenytoin
- ❏ B phenobarbitone
- ❏ C cimetidine
- ❏ D carbamazepine
- ❏ E metronidazole

1.12 Cytochrome P450 is

- ❏ A found in lysosomes
- ❏ B found in hepatocytes
- ❏ C found in the endoplasmic reticulum
- ❏ D found in the mitochondria
- ❏ E responsible for the oxidation and reduction of drugs

1.13 pH alters the structure of

- ❏ A atracurium
- ❏ B midazolam
- ❏ C diazepam
- ❏ D suxamethonium
- ❏ E morphine

1.14 Metoclopramide causes

- ❏ A increased prolactin secretion
- ❏ B hypertension
- ❏ C oculogyric crisis
- ❏ D increased lower oesophageal tone
- ❏ E nausea

1.15 Reduction in uterine tone is caused by

- ❑ A halothane
- ❑ B amyl nitrate
- ❑ C β-adrenoreceptor agonists
- ❑ D neostigmine
- ❑ E labetalol

1.16 Rate of transfer across the placenta depends upon

- ❑ A the size of the molecule
- ❑ B the lipid solubility of the molecule
- ❑ C the blood flow to the placenta
- ❑ D the duration of the pregnancy
- ❑ E the fetal haemoglobin

1.17 The following cause a reduction in the cerebrovascular resistance

- ❑ A enflurane
- ❑ B thiopentone
- ❑ C ether
- ❑ D isoflurane
- ❑ E fentanyl

1.18 The following contaminants of nitrous oxide cause pulmonary oedema

- ❑ A nitric oxide
- ❑ B nitrogen dioxide
- ❑ C ammonia
- ❑ D carbon monoxide
- ❑ E nitrogen

1.19 Nifedipine

- ❑ A causes tremor
- ❑ B causes increased cardiac output
- ❑ C causes vasodilatation
- ❑ D is not absorbed orally
- ❑ E is synergistic in its action with halothane

1.20 Ropivacaine

- ❏ A is a racemic mixture
- ❏ B is less cardiotoxic than bupivacaine
- ❏ C is more potent than bupivacaine
- ❏ D has the same pKa as bupivacaine
- ❏ E produces greater motor block than bupivacaine

1.21 With regard to magnesium

- ❏ A it is an anticonvulsant
- ❏ B it is a neuromuscular blocking drug
- ❏ C it causes cardiac arrhythmias
- ❏ D the normal plasma level is 1 mmol/l
- ❏ E the plasma level is controlled by calcitonin

1.22 Isoflurane

- ❏ A reduces systemic vascular resistance
- ❏ B reduces cardiac output
- ❏ C reduces stroke volume
- ❏ D causes a dose-dependent drop in blood pressure
- ❏ E increases heart rate

1.23 Propofol

- ❏ A is dissolved in propylene glycol
- ❏ B is metabolised in the liver
- ❏ C causes less respiratory depression than thiopentone
- ❏ D reduces the blood pressure
- ❏ E has a pH of 7

1.24 The following have anticonvulsant activity

- ❏ A clonazepam
- ❏ B thiopentone
- ❏ C phenytoin
- ❏ D ketamine
- ❏ E propofol

1.25 Suxamethonium

- ❏ A causes a decrease in heart rate in repeated doses
- ❏ B competes with procaine for acetylcholinesterase
- ❏ C prolongs subsequent block with atracurium
- ❏ D is effective and painless by the intramuscular route
- ❏ E is stable in solution

1.26 Vecuronium

- ❏ A is a monoquaternary amine
- ❏ B inhibits noradrenaline re-uptake at clinical doses
- ❏ C provides as effective a block as suxamethonium at 60 seconds
- ❏ D has a dose-dependent duration of action
- ❏ E is dependent on renal excretion

1.27 Ketamine

- ❏ A reduces bronchial secretions
- ❏ B is dangerous in patients with angina
- ❏ C is dangerous in patients with asthma
- ❏ D is stable in solution
- ❏ E is excreted unchanged in the urine

1.28 Atenolol is

- ❏ A a non-selective beta antagonist
- ❏ B safe in asthmatics
- ❏ C safe in renal failure
- ❏ D safe in diabetics
- ❏ E a negative inotrope

1.29 The half-life of lidocaine is increased by

- ❏ A increasing age
- ❏ B plasma acetylcholinesterase
- ❏ C propranolol
- ❏ D phenobarbitone
- ❏ E haemorrhagic shock

1.30 Amiodarone

- ❏ A is a hydroxy quinolone compound
- ❏ B can cause hypoparathyroidism in long-term administration
- ❏ C is associated with corneal deposits
- ❏ D is used to treat supraventricular tachycardia in the presence of adrenergic blockade
- ❏ E has a half-life of 9 hours

1.31 The following electrolyte changes occur

- ❏ A hypocalcaemia with hyperparathyroidism
- ❏ B hypercalcaemia with acute pancreatitis
- ❏ C hypoglycaemia with phaeochromocytoma
- ❏ . D hyperkalaemia with malignant hyperpyrexia
- ❏ E hyponatraemia with TURP syndrome

1.32 Physiological changes in pregnancy include

- ❏ A an increase in functional residual capacity
- ❏ B the oxyhaemoglobin dissociation curve is shifted to the left
- ❏ C anaemia, which is usually due to a fall in red cell mass
- ❏ D increased lower oesophageal sphincter tone
- ❏ E an increase in systemic vascular resistance

1.33 Regarding bleeding disorders

- ❏ A bleeding is likely when the platelet count reaches a level of $140 \times 10^9/l$
- ❏ B bleeding time is increased in haemophilia
- ❏ C excessive bleeding following multiple transfusions with stored blood or large volumes of crystalloid is mainly due to deficiency of platelets and factors V and VIII
- ❏ D all coagulation proteins are synthesised by the liver and require vitamin K for their synthesis
- ❏ E bleeding due to excessive warfarin is rapidly corrected by vitamin K

1.34 Regarding deep vein thrombosis (DVT)

❑   A   the incidence of DVT has not fallen despite the use of prophylactic anti-thrombotic measures

❑   B   the treatment of small post-operative pulmonary embolism is thrombolytic therapy (eg streptokinase)

❑   C   the risk of DVT is higher with knee and hip operations than with other surgical procedures

❑   D   epidurals and spinals are absolutely contraindicated in patients receiving prophylactic subcutaneous heparin

❑   E   it is advisable to discontinue hormone replacement therapy (HRT) in women undergoing an elective surgical procedure

1.35 A 30-year-old man has the following blood gas analysis breathing air: pH 7.54, PaO_2 55 mmHg (7.2 kPa), $PaCO_2$ 25 mmHg (3.3 kPa). The following conditions could account for such results

❑   A   carbon monoxide poisoning

❑   B   ascent to high altitude

❑   C   spontaneous pneumothorax

❑   D   hysteria

❑   E   salicylate poisoning

1.36 Acute hypovolaemia leads to the following physiological changes

❑   A   increased physiological dead space

❑   B   hypoxaemia

❑   C   raised arterial $PaCO_2$

❑   D   increased renal blood flow

❑   E   increased alveolar-to-arterial oxygen gradient

1.37 A bleeding disorder in which there is no clot retraction could be due to deficiency of

❑   A   platelets

❑   B   prothrombin

❑   C   calcium ions

❑   D   fibrinogen

❑   E   vitamin K

1.38 An increased arterial $PaCO_2$ is associated with

- ❏ A increased adrenaline release
- ❏ B tachycardia
- ❏ C hypertension
- ❏ D increased catecholamine release
- ❏ E increased sweating

1.39 A Valsalva manoeuvre

- ❏ A is a forced expiration against a closed glottis or other airway obstruction
- ❏ B is initially associated with increased systolic arterial pressure
- ❏ C is associated with decreased peripheral resistance
- ❏ D is normally associated with a tachycardia
- ❏ E is normally associated with a bradycardia

1.40 Albumin

- ❏ A has a molecular weight of approximately 65,000 Da
- ❏ B is increased in liver disease
- ❏ C is increased in malabsorption syndrome
- ❏ D makes a significant contribution to plasma oncotic pressure
- ❏ E has a normal value of 34–45 g/l

1.41 The minute volume is

- ❏ A reduced during sleep
- ❏ B reduced by a rise in body temperature
- ❏ C reduced by an increase in body acidity
- ❏ D increased in hypothermia
- ❏ E increased by arrival at an altitude of 5000 m

1.42 The haemoglobin–oxygen dissociation curve is moved to the right by

- ❏ A acidosis
- ❏ B raised body temperature
- ❏ C an increase in body acidity
- ❏ D ageing
- ❏ E anaemia

1.43 In the normal heart

❑ A blood in the left atrium contains less oxygen than the blood in the pulmonary artery
❑ B right ventricular pressure might be 25/10 mmHg
❑ C pulmonary artery systolic pressure is usually about 10 mmHg less than right ventricular systolic pressure
❑ D left ventricular pressure might be 125/8 mmHg
❑ E blood in the pulmonary artery has an oxygen saturation of 75%

1.44 Transmitters at the autonomic ganglia include

❑ A 5-HT
❑ B glycine
❑ C acetylcholine
❑ D butylcholine
❑ E noradrenaline

1.45 Reabsorption of sodium in the kidney

❑ A is regulated by ADH
❑ B occurs in the proximal tubule
❑ C occurs by active transport in the loop of Henle
❑ D is influenced by Starling's forces
❑ E is associated with chloride reabsorption

1.46 Block of the cervical sympathetic ganglia causes

❑ A dilatation of the conjunctival vessels
❑ B anhidrosis of the ipsilateral face
❑ C miosis
❑ D nasal congestion
❑ E enophthalmos

1.47 Metabolic acidosis can be caused by

❑ A a pancreatic fistula
❑ B hypoventilation
❑ C severe diarrhoea
❑ D renal failure
❑ E transplantation of the ureters into the colon

1.48 Results of prolonged severe vomiting, complicating pyloric stenosis, include

- ❏ A hyperchloraemia
- ❏ B impaired renal bicarbonate excretion
- ❏ C hyperventilation
- ❏ D acidic urine excretion
- ❏ E hypokalaemia

1.49 Regarding ABO blood groups

- ❏ A they are an example of Mendelian dominant inheritance
- ❏ B they may be detected in saliva
- ❏ C they are independent of Rhesus blood groups
- ❏ D AB blood can be given to A and B recipients
- ❏ E O-negative blood can be given to anyone

1.50 The following are likely to occur in the first 10 minutes of accidental insertion of the endotracheal tube into the right main bronchus

- ❏ A arterial hypotension
- ❏ B severe hypercapnia
- ❏ C apparent increase in inhalation anaesthetic requirement
- ❏ D increased inflation pressure
- ❏ E collapse of the right upper lobe

1.51 The normal arterial pH

- ❏ A has a hydrogen ion concentration of 40 mmol/l
- ❏ B is maintained by excreting approximately 60 mmol of hydrogen ions per day
- ❏ C is calculated from the measured PCO_2 and bicarbonate in blood gas analysers
- ❏ D is maintained principally by intracellular buffering systems
- ❏ E is slightly higher in the neonate than in the adult

1.52 In the normal ECG

- [ ] A the PR interval is the total time for actual polarisation
- [ ] B the QT interval measures less than 0.44 s
- [ ] C the normal PR interval is 0.06–1 s
- [ ] D a QRS complex duration greater than 0.1 s equals a conduction delay
- [ ] E the ST interval is the time for ventricular repolarisation

1.53 When calculating lung volumes

- [ ] A the anatomical dead space may be estimated using the Bohr equation
- [ ] B the V_d/V_t is normally 0.3 at rest
- [ ] C the FRC cannot be measured directly
- [ ] D changes in expired nitrogen concentration may be used to determine closing volume
- [ ] E changes in expired nitrogen concentration may be used to determine residual volume

1.54 When measuring glomerular filtration rate (GFR)

- [ ] A renal blood flow must be measured or estimated
- [ ] B the indicator substance used must not undergo reabsorption following tubular excretion
- [ ] C the result matches the clearance of the indicator if it is really inert
- [ ] D using sodium as an indicator gives an erroneously high GFR
- [ ] E the average value for an adult male would be 125 ml/min

1.55 With regard to basal metabolic rate (BMR)

- [ ] A BMR is the energy output of the individual at rest at room temperature
- [ ] B for every 1°C rise in body temperature, the BMR increases by 8%
- [ ] C carbohydrates stimulate BMR more than proteins
- [ ] D BMR increases with age
- [ ] E BMR is higher in males than in females

1.56 Regarding total parenteral nutrition (TPN)

- [ ] A the entire calorific requirement can be provided by glucose
- [ ] B daily nitrogen requirements are greater in the elderly than in the young patient
- [ ] C amino acids are provided as dextro isomers
- [ ] D the use of enteral feeding is associated with a lower infection rate
- [ ] E glutamine is available in most commercial amino acid preparations

1.57 The measurement of cardiac output by thermodilution

- [ ] A is accurate and easily repeatable
- [ ] B involves measuring the integral of temperature change over time
- [ ] C involves use of the latent heat of vaporisation in the calculations
- [ ] D is also known as the Fick technique
- [ ] E may be inaccurate due to respiratory changes in the pulmonary artery temperature

1.58 Regarding the Glasgow Coma Scale

- [ ] A it acts as a guide to the severity of a head injury
- [ ] B it is a prognostic guide
- [ ] C a score of 2 is incompatible with survival
- [ ] D if the patient's best motor response to pain is flexion, this adds 3 to the total score
- [ ] E it is useless in paediatric patients

1.59 When measuring central venous pressure (CVP)

- [ ] A +5 mmHg is higher than +5 mmH$_2$O
- [ ] B CVP is a reliable indicator of left ventricular function
- [ ] C the catheter should be in the right atrium
- [ ] D a normal CVP excludes the diagnosis of pulmonary oedema
- [ ] E the value of the CVP measurement is unaffected by therapeutic vasoconstriction

1.60 Pulse oximetry

- ❑ A gives a falsely low reading in the presence of tricuspid incompetence
- ❑ B is designed to measure light absorption every 0.5 s
- ❑ C gives a rapid response to changes in alveolar gas tensions
- ❑ D light measurement comes from a filtered light source
- ❑ E can give a falsely high reading in heavy smokers due to the carboxyhaemoglobin concentration

1.61 In an explosion

- ❑ A the speed of reaction is greatest with a stoichiometric concentration
- ❑ B the reaction is more vigorous with oxygen than with nitrous oxide
- ❑ C 1 microjoule of energy is sufficient for reactions in oxygen
- ❑ D the likelihood of sparking is reduced by keeping the relative humidity greater than 50% and the temperature more than 20°C
- ❑ E the stoichiometric concentration of a fuel and oxidising agent is the concentration at which an explosion occurs

1.62 When assessing neuromuscular blockade

- ❑ A double burst stimulation is of particular value when there is no train of four present
- ❑ B double burst stimulation is two short tetanic stimuli 750 ms apart
- ❑ C train of four stimulation consists of 4 pulses at 2 Hz
- ❑ D a fading pattern of train of four excludes prolongation of suxamethonium
- ❑ E use of facial nerve overestimates the degree of neuromuscular blockade

1.63 With regard to diathermy

- ❑ A it uses an alternating current of 0.5–1 mHz
- ❑ B a sine wave pattern is used for cutting
- ❑ C it can act as an ignition source for bowel gas
- ❑ D bipolar diathermy requires the use of a diathermy plate
- ❑ E bipolar diathermy is safer in patients with pacemakers

1.64 Measures taken to minimise heat loss during surgery include

- ❏ A operating theatre temperature at 20°C
- ❏ B giving fluids into central vein
- ❏ C humidifying inspired gases
- ❏ D small doses of phenothiazines
- ❏ E the use of space blankets

1.65 The following may lead to the over-estimation of blood pressure

- ❏ A using too wide a cuff
- ❏ B a fat arm in a standard cuff
- ❏ C letting the cuff down too slowly
- ❏ D having the sphygmomanometer above the patient
- ❏ E severe atherosclerosis

1.66 The saturated vapour pressure of a liquid

- ❏ A is linearly related to temperature
- ❏ B can exceed the normal atmospheric pressure
- ❏ C is a function of barometric pressure
- ❏ D for isoflurane is around 32 kPa at 20°C
- ❏ E is 7.6 kPa for water at 37°C

1.67 For laminar flow in a tube, the flow rate is directly proportional to

- ❏ A its length
- ❏ B the fourth power of its radius
- ❏ C the density of the gas or liquid flowing through it
- ❏ D the pressure drop across it
- ❏ E the viscosity of the gas or liquid flowing across it

1.68 Helium has the following advantages over nitrogen for divers at depth

- ❏ A it diffuses more rapidly into the body tissues
- ❏ B it is denser
- ❏ C it has a lower viscosity
- ❏ D it has less narcotic effect
- ❏ E it is a good insulator

1.69 In a recording of central venous pressure (CVP)

- ❏ A the a wave is caused by atrial systole
- ❏ B the c wave is caused by bulging of the tricuspid valve during isometric ventricular contraction
- ❏ C the v wave is due to atrial filling when the tricuspid valve is closed
- ❏ D the pressure wave is increased during inspiration
- ❏ E the pressure wave is always raised if left atrial pressure is increased

1.70 Soda lime

- ❏ A is mainly calcium carbonate
- ❏ B can be used to scavenge nitrous oxide
- ❏ C needs water to absorb carbon dioxide
- ❏ D when in a properly packed canister, half the volume should be space between granules
- ❏ E gets hot in use

1.71 Warming blood to 37°C for massive blood transfusion

- ❏ A reduces the incidence of infection
- ❏ B increases the CO_2 tension
- ❏ C reduces the O_2 tension
- ❏ D shifts the O_2 dissociation curve to the right
- ❏ E reduces the incidence of arrhythmias

1.72 Concerning fires and explosions in theatre

- ❏ A the relative humidity in theatre should be about 66%
- ❏ B air is safer than oxygen
- ❏ C switches in the zone of risk should be spark proof
- ❏ D the floor should be terrazzo on a well-conducting screed
- ❏ E cotton fabrics are better than wool

1.73 Critical temperature

- ❏ A of nitrous oxide is 36.5°C
- ❏ B is the temperature below which a gas cannot be liquefied by pressure
- ❏ C separates gases from vapours
- ❏ D of O_2 is –182.5°C
- ❏ E is always lower than the boiling point of the same gas

1.74 The following are true for gases in cylinders

- ❏ A nitrous oxide and Entonox are filled to the same pressure
- ❏ B a full oxygen cylinder is at a pressure of 1950 kPa
- ❏ C nitrous oxide should contain 1% water vapour
- ❏ D nitrous oxide should not be stored below –8°C
- ❏ E size E cylinders of oxygen and nitrous oxide are generally used on a Boyle's machine

1.75 With regard to pressure

- ❏ A it is measured in newtons
- ❏ B it is defined as the force applied over a surface
- ❏ C the absolute pressure of a cylinder of O_2 is 138 bar
- ❏ D arterial blood pressure readings are gauge pressures
- ❏ E when using a narrow capillary tube filled with water to measure pressure, the reading will be decreased due to the effect of surface tension

1.76 Regarding turbulent flow

- ❏ A the flow is directly proportional to pressure
- ❏ B the flow is directly proportional to the density of the fluid
- ❏ C its onset can be predicted by a Reynolds' number greater than 1000
- ❏ D warming anaesthetic gases increases the likelihood of turbulent flow
- ❏ E this is more likely in the lower respiratory tract

1.77 Regarding the gas laws

- ❑ A at constant temperature, the volume of a given mass of gas varies directly with the absolute pressure
- ❑ B at constant pressure, the volume of a given mass of gas varies directly with the temperature
- ❑ C at a constant volume, the temperature of a given mass of gas varies directly with the absolute pressure
- ❑ D in a mixture of gases, the partial pressure that each gas exerts is dependent on the constituent mixture
- ❑ E alteration of the state of a gas without allowing the temperature to alter is known as an antidiabetic change

1.78 The critical temperature

- ❑ A is the temperature below which a substance cannot be liquefied by pressure alone
- ❑ B of oxygen is −119°C
- ❑ C of nitrous oxide is 36.5°C
- ❑ D applies only to a single gas, not a mixture
- ❑ E of CO_2 is 31°C

1.79 Concerning humidification

- ❑ A inspired gases in the trachea contain approximately 3 mg of water vapour per litre of dry gas, if dry gas has been inhaled
- ❑ B humidification of inspired gases results in less heat loss than warming inspired gases
- ❑ C the heat moisture exchanger (HME) can give a humidity of the inspired gases of about 20 g/m³
- ❑ D the HME is more efficient and more effective as the ambient temperature increases
- ❑ E using the HME can increase the work of breathing

1.80 The following can be used for the measurement of temperature

- ❑ A the Seebeck effect
- ❑ B alcohol thermometers
- ❑ C mercury thermometers
- ❑ D resistance
- ❑ E interferometer

1.81 A Wright's respirometer will give a reading which is lower than the actual value when there is

❏ A low flow of gas
❏ B 30% oxygen in the gas
❏ C nitrous oxide present
❏ D humidity in the respirometer
❏ E an intermittent flow of gas

1.82 Evoked potential techniques for measuring depth of anaesthesia utilise the following stimuli

❏ A auditory
❏ B oesophageal contractions
❏ C somatosensory
❏ D visual
❏ E magnetic resonance

1.83 In exponential change

❏ A the time constant is the time taken for the initial response to fall to half its value
❏ B in one time constant, 37% change is complete
❏ C in three time constants, 95% change is complete
❏ D the rate of change of a variable is proportional to the magnitude of the variable
❏ E the half-life is the time constant

1.84 Airway resistance

❏ A can be measured by plethysmography
❏ B is measured in kPa per litre
❏ C increases during inhalation anaesthesia
❏ D increases at high inspiratory flow rates
❏ E decreases with the application of positive end expiratory pressure

1.85 The chances of microshock occurring increases due to

- ❑ A saline-filled catheters
- ❑ B earth loop
- ❑ C multiple earth connections
- ❑ D isolated circuit
- ❑ E oesophageal electrocardiogram

1.86 The following are required to measure the cardiac output by the Fick principle

- ❑ A arterial oxygen content
- ❑ B venous oxygen content
- ❑ C oxygen uptake
- ❑ D respiratory quotient
- ❑ E arterial carbon monoxide content

1.87 Regarding the Magill circuit

- ❑ A it is an example of a Mapleson A circuit
- ❑ B it is functionally similar to the Lack circuit
- ❑ C it is suitable for children over 25 kg
- ❑ D it is suitable for IPPV
- ❑ E during spontaneous ventilation rebreathing and hypercarbia will occur if the fresh gas flow is less than the minute volume

1.88 Inaccuracies in the measurement of central venous pressure may arise from

- ❑ A a change in the position of the patient
- ❑ B misplacement of the catheter
- ❑ C wetting of the cotton wool plug in the top of the manometer tube
- ❑ D straining during respiration
- ❑ E arterial hypotension

1.89 The accuracy of a rotameter may be affected by

- ❑ A dirt on the bobbin
- ❑ B static electricity
- ❑ C passing the wrong gas through it
- ❑ D back pressure from the Manley ventilator
- ❑ E using it at high altitude

1.90 Regarding capnography

❏   A   it works on the absorption of carbon dioxide in the ultra violet region of the spectrum

❏   B   it can be helpful in detecting air embolism before cardiovascular compromise occurs

❏   C   the P_aCO_2/P_eCO_2 gradient in a patient with V/Q mismatch is 0.7 kPa

❏   D   collision broadening may occur in the presence of oxygen

❏   E   the two sampling methods are side and main stream

MCQ Paper 1 – Answers

1.1   Answers: C E

Dopamine is both a catecholamine and a neurotransmitter. It is positively inotropic and chronotropic and may cause tachyarrhythmias. It causes renal artery dilatation. Dopamine is also an important neurotransmitter in the central nervous system, particularly in the basal ganglia. A deficiency of dopaminergic neurones in the basal ganglia causes Parkinsonism. Dopamine acts to inhibit prolactin secretion by the posterior pituitary gland. Finally, dopamine is the neurotransmitter at the chemoreceptor trigger zone. From the above information, it can be deduced that dopamine antagonists might cause extrapyramidal effects such as Parkinsonism and oculogyric crises. They may cause hyperprolactinaemia. Their principal use is as anti-emetics. The commonly encountered dopamine antagonists include the phenothiazines such as prochlorperazine and chlorpromazine, butyrophenones such as haloperidol, and others such as metoclopramide.

As well as its anti-emetic effects, metoclopramide usefully raises lower oesophageal sphincter tone and promotes gastric emptying. These effects are due to cholinergic (not anti-dopaminergic) effects, however. Metoclopramide also has anti-serotoninergic effects.

1.2   Answers: C D E

Diamorphine is diacetyl morphine, it is rapidly metabolised in the liver to the active metabolites monoacetylmorphine and, ultimately, morphine. It is therefore a pro-drug with a high first-pass metabolism. It is about twice as potent as morphine and is more rapid in action because of greater lipid solubility. Diamorphine is more euphoric and a better antitussive than morphine.

1.3   Answers: D E

Alfentanil is about one-tenth as potent as fentanyl. The pKa of alfentanil is 6.5, whereas that of fentanyl is 8.4. Thus, at physiological pH, 89% of alfentanil is in the unionised form, whilst only 9% of fentanyl is unionised. Since it is the unionised form that crosses cell membranes, alfentanil acts much faster than fentanyl, despite being less lipid soluble. Alfentanil has a smaller volume of distribution and a shorter elimination half-life, and its duration of action is thus shorter than that of fentanyl. Alfentanil has minimal cardiovascular effects, although it may cause bradycardia and hypotension. Both drugs may cause muscle chest wall rigidity which may be so severe as to make artificial ventilation very difficult.

1.4 Answers: B D

Methohexitone is a methylated oxybarbiturate; the drug is reconstituted to make a 1% solution (10 mg/ml) which has a pH of 11. It is used mainly in electroconvulsive therapy and dental anaesthesia. Although it is a barbiturate, it may cause convulsions in epileptics and may precipitate porphyria. The usual dose in an adult is 1–2 mg/kg compared with 3–6 mg/kg for thiopentone. Both methohexitone and thiopentone are 80% bound to plasma proteins.

1.5 Answers: A B E

Propofol is 2,6-disopropylphenol. It is presented as a 1% white emulsion (10 mg/ml). The emulsion consists of 10% soya bean oil, 1.2% purified egg phosphatide and 2.25% glycerol. Propofol causes greater hypotension than thiopentone, mainly by vasodilatation; it also causes greater respiratory depression than thiopentone. The induction dose in an adult is 1.5–2.5 mg/kg. It is metabolised in the liver and other extra-hepatic sites such as the lungs.

1.6 Answers: B C D E

Non-depolarising neuromuscular block is characterised by fade and post-tetanic facilitation, whilst fasciculation occurs with the depolarising drugs such as suxamethonium. Non-depolarising muscle relaxant drugs are reversed by acetylcholinesterase inhibitors such as neostigmine. Neostigmine exacerbates block by a depolarising agent. The effects of non-depolarising agents are prolonged by hypothermia, hypokalaemia, hypocalcaemia and hypermagnesaemia, aminoglycosides and myasthenia gravis.

Metabolic acidosis prolongs the effect of some, but not all, non-depolarising muscle relaxants.

1.7 Answers: A B C E

Atracurium is a non-depolarising muscle relaxant of the benzylisoquinolinium group. The other main group of relaxant drugs is the aminosteroids which include vecuronium. Atracurium is a mixture of ten isomers. *cis*-Atracurium is the *R-cis R1-cis* isomer of atracurium. Atracurium comes as a 1% solution (10 mg/ml), the adult dose is about 0.5 mg/kg. Atracurium is broken down by Hoffman degradation (which is temperature dependent) and alkaline ester hydrolysis. The former reaction produces laudanosine, which causes seizures in dogs but seems harmless to humans. Hypothermia and acidosis prolong the action of atracurium. Atracurium can cause histamine release.

1.8 Answers: A E

Inotropic agents increase the force of contraction of the myocardium. Such agents include the catecholamines (such as dopamine, adrenaline and noradrenaline) which act by stimulating β-adrenergic receptors in the myocardium. Phosphodiesterase inhibitors (such as the theophyllines) act by blocking the breakdown of cAMP. cAMP is the second messenger which is produced by β-adrenergic receptor stimulation.

Glucagon is a positive inotrope which acts by stimulating the activity of adenylate cyclase, leading to an increase in intracellular concentrations of cAMP. Verapamil, propranolol and potassium all have negative inotropic effects.

1.9 Answers: A D E

Many drugs are metabolised in the liver. The cytochrome P450 enzyme system is the major metabolic route. Most drugs are metabolised to more water-soluble compounds which can then be renally excreted.

Hepatic metabolism usually involves two steps:
phase 1 – oxidation, reduction, hydrolysis (cytochrome P450)
phase 2 – conjugation with either glucuronide or by glycine, glutathione, sulphate, acetyl or methyl groups

1.10 Answers: A B C D E

Bupivacaine is an amide local anaesthetic agent. All amides have the same basic structure (see overleaf):

Amide functional group

Bupivacaine has a longer duration of action than lignocaine and is more potent (0.25% bupivacaine is equipotent with 1% lignocaine).

Bupivacaine is cardiotoxic and is contraindicated in intravenous regional anaesthesia (IVRA; Bier's block).

Prilocaine is the agent of choice for IVRA. It is thought that the cardiotoxicity is due to the D stereoisomer. The pure L enantiomer (laevo-bupivacaine) has been developed to overcome this problem.

Ropivacaine has the same chemical structure as bupivacaine, but has one extra carbon atom in the amine R1 group. It is less cardiotoxic and may preferentially block sensory rather than motor fibres.

1.11 Answers: A B D

1.12 Answers: B C E

The cytochrome P450 enzyme system is found in the endoplasmic reticulum of hepatocytes and is responsible for phase 1 metabolic reactions such as oxidation and reduction. The enzyme system can be induced or inhibited by drugs. Enzyme induction can lead to reduced plasma levels of drugs which undergo hepatic cytochrome P450 metabolism leading to a reduced pharmacological effect. Alcohol is the most commonly found enzyme inducer in the general public. Rifampicin is an enzyme-inducing agent which may reduce the efficacy of drugs, eg warfarin or the oral contraceptive pill, which undergo hepatic cytochrome P450 metabolism. Conversely, inhibition of cytochrome P450 (by cimetidine for example) can lead to toxic levels of drugs such as phenytoin or warfarin.

P450 Induction	P450 Inhibition
Barbiturates	Cimetidine
Rifampicin	
Phenytoin &	
other anticonvulsants	

1.13 Answers: A B

Midazolam is presented as a solution with a pH < 4. On entering venous blood, the pH increases and the structure of the molecule changes in such a way as to render it active. Atracurium undergoes spontaneous Hoffman degradation (which is both temperature and pH dependent); its structure changes with pH.

1.14 Answers: A C D

Metoclopramide is a dopamine antagonist which is used as an anti-emetic.

It also raises lower oesophageal sphincter tone. Like other anti-dopaminergic drugs, it may cause extrapyramidal effects such as oculogyric crises, especially in the young.

Since dopamine is a prolactin inhibiting factor, drugs that are anti-dopaminergic can cause hyperprolactinaemia.

1.15 Answers: A B C

Uterine smooth muscle has sympathetic and parasympathetic innervation. Sympathetic stimulation by $\beta2$-adrenoreceptor agonists such as salbutamol or ritodrine relaxes the uterus; whilst parasympathetic stimulation causes contraction. Neostigmine, by inhibiting acetylcholinesterase, has parasympathomimetic effects.

Amyl nitrate and halothane directly relax smooth muscle. Oxytocin and its analogues are potent uterine contractors.

1.16 Answers: A B C

The rate of transfer of a molecule across the placenta is indirectly proportional to its size and directly related to its lipid solubility.

Clearly, the blood flow to the placenta is important too.

1.17 Answers: A C D

All the volatile agents cause a reduction in cerebrovascular resistance. Thiopentone and fentanyl cause little change.

1.18 Answers: A B C

Nitrous oxide (N_2O) may be contaminated by nitric oxide (NO) and nitrogen dioxide (NO_2) produced during the manufacture of nitrous oxide. The higher oxides of nitrogen can produce pulmonary oedema several hours after inhalation, and pulmonary fibrosis 2–3 weeks later. They may also cause methaemoglobinaemia. Nitrous oxide is manufactured by heating ammonium nitrate to 240°C. Ammonia is produced in this reaction and may contaminate nitrous oxide. It too can cause pulmonary oedema.

1.19 Answer: B C

Nifedipine is a calcium channel blocking drug used to treat hypertension. It is a vasodilator, causing an increase in cardiac output, due to the vasodilatation and a fall in the systemic vascular resistance, hypotension and reflex tachycardia. It may be taken orally or sublingually and may cause headache, flushing, dizziness and peripheral oedema.

1.20 Answers: B D

Ropivacaine is a amide local anaesthetic agent. It is less potent than bupivacaine, but has a similar duration of action. It causes less central nervous system and cardiovascular toxicity than bupivacaine and, in addition, less motor block. It is presented as the pure S enantiomer, not a racemic mixture. Bupivacaine is a racemic mixture; the pure enantiomer is now available commercially. The pKa values of ropivacaine and bupivacaine are identical.

1.21 Answers: A B D

Magnesium is the second most plentiful intracellular cation after potassium, and is one of the most important regulators of intracellular biochemistry. The normal plasma level is 0.75–1.0 mmol/l. Magnesium is used therapeutically to control cardiac arrhythmias and as an anticonvulsant in eclampsia. Magnesium toxicity causes neuromuscular blockade by inhibiting acetylcholine release at the neuromuscular junction. The primary clinical manifestation of this is respiratory depression and loss of tendon reflexes. Treatment is intravenous calcium gluconate. Magnesium is controlled by parathormone, but not by calcitonin.

1.22 Answers: A B C D E

Isoflurane causes a small (10%) drop in cardiac output in healthy volunteers, mainly by a decrease in stroke volume. Isoflurane causes significant peripheral vasodilatation and hypotension with a reflex compensatory tachycardia.

1.23 Answers: B D E

Propofol is presented as a white aqueous emulsion containing 10% soya bean oil, 2.25% glycerol and 1.2% purified egg phosphatide.

It has a pH of 7 and a pKa of 11. It causes more respiratory depression and greater hypotension than thiopentone. It is metabolised in the liver as well as at other extra-hepatic sites.

1.24 Answers: A B C E

Benzodiazepines are $GABA_A$ receptor antagonists, and barbiturates enhance $GABA_A$-mediated inhibition of postsynaptic neurones. Phenytoin inhibits neuronal sodium channels. Propofol enhances $GABA_A$ activity, and has been used successfully in intractable epilepsy.

1.25 Answer: A

Suxamethonium is a depolarising neuromuscular blocking agent. It is stored at 4°C in the fridge, although its potency in fact decreases very slowly if left at room temperature. Chemically, suxamethonium is two molecules of acetylcholine linked by ester bonds. The ester bonds are broken down by plasma cholinesterase. The productivity of this enzyme is controlled genetically by at least five alleles. A proportion of the population have atypical plasma cholinesterase and metabolise the drug more slowly than normal. Low levels of plasma cholinesterase are found in patients undergoing plasmapheresis, in liver failure, in malnutrition, during pregnancy, and in patients taking the oral contraceptive pill, lithium or cyclophosphamide. The side-effects of suxamethonium include:

hyperkalaemia, muscle pains and bradycardia; especially with repeat doses. Suxamethonium may be given intramuscularly but it is painful.

1.26 Answers: A D

Vecuronium is a non-depolarising muscle relaxant. It is a monoquaternary aminosteroid, becoming bisquaternary at pH 7.4. It acts in about 2 minutes and has a duration of action of about 20–30 minutes. It is devoid of cardio-vascular actions and is metabolised in the liver to inactive products.

1.27 Answers: B D

Ketamine is a phencyclidine derivative. It produces a state known as dissociative anaesthesia. Its mode of action includes antagonism at the N-methyl-D-aspartate (NMDA) receptor as well as actions at the adrenergic, cholinergic, serotoninergic and opioid receptors. It is a potent analgesic as well as being a bronchodilator and sympathomimetic agent. It is thus useful in asthmatic and shocked patients, but contraindicated in angina and hypertension. It causes hypersalivation and increased bronchial secretions. An antisialogogue pre-medication is often therefore used with ketamine. It raises intraocular and intracranial pressure and may produce disturbing emergence reactions. It undergoes hepatic metabolism and renal excretion; only 2.5% is excreted unchanged in the urine.

1.28 Answer: E

Atenolol is a relatively selective antagonist at the β1-receptors.

Despite this, it is not entirely safe in asthmatics as blockade of β2-receptors may precipitate bronchospasm. Like all beta blockers, atenolol is a negative inotrope and may be unsafe in diabetics as it may mask the sympathetic symptoms of hypoglycaemia, such as sweating and tachycardia. Atenolol is renally excreted and should not be used in patients with renal failure as it will accumulate.

1.29 Answers: C E

Lidocaine is an amide local anaesthetic which is highly protein bound (65%). It undergoes hepatic metabolism by amidases, unlike the ester local anaes-thetics, such as cocaine, which are degraded by plasma cholinesterase. It undergoes extensive first pass metabolism (70%). The half-life of lidocaine is increased in haemorrhagic shock because of reduced hepatic blood flow, and therefore a reduced rate of metabolism. Propranolol decreases the clearance of amide local anaesthetic agents by decreasing hepatic blood flow and therefore reducing the rate of metabolism.

1.30 Answers: C D

Amiodarone is in class III of the Vaughan-Williams' classification of anti-arrhythmics. It is used to treat both ventricular and supraventricular arrhythmias. It has a number of side-effects, including a photosensitive slate-grey skin discoloration and reversible corneal microdeposits. It is an iodine-containing compound, and can therefore interfere with thyroid function. It can cause hypo- or hyperthyroidism. It can cause pulmonary fibrosis, hepatic dysfunction and peripheral neuropathy. It has a very long half-life.

1.31 Answers: D E

Hypercalcaemia occurs in hyperparathyroidism. Hypocalcaemia occurs in hypoparathyroidism and also in acute pancreatitis.

Hyperglycaemia is seen in phaeochromocytoma due to high levels of catecholamines. Malignant hyperpyrexia leads to muscle breakdown, release of intracellular potassium and hyperkalaemia.

The TURP syndrome is caused by excessive absorption of irrigation fluid into the vascular space and leads to hyponatraemia.

1.32 Answer: All false

In pregnancy, there are great physiological changes.
- The circulation is hyperdynamic with a reduced systemic vascular resistance and an increase in heart rate, stroke volume and cardiac output.
- Although there is an increase in red cell mass, there is an even greater increase in plasma volume leading to the physiological anaemia of pregnancy.
- The oxygen dissociation curve shifts to the right, thus facilitating oxygen uptake by the fetal red cells.
- In the respiratory system, there is a reduction in functional residual capacity, but an increased tidal volume and respiratory rate.
- There is an increase in fibrinogen and reduced fibrinolysis leading to a hypercoagulable state.
- The lower oesophageal sphincter tone is reduced in pregnancy leading to an increased likelihood of gastric reflux. It is because of this that pregnant women having a general anaesthetic are given sodium citrate and ranitidine and have a rapid sequence induction with cricoid pressure to reduce the chance of regurgitation and aspiration of acidic stomach contents.

1.33 Answer: C

Bleeding is unlikely until the platelet count falls to $50\times10^9/l$ and may not occur until an even lower level. Haemophilia is an X-linked disorder in which there is a deficiency of factor VIII. It results in a prolongation of the aPTT. The PT, platelet count and bleeding time are all normal. Stored blood contains no functional platelets and is deficient in the labile clotting factors (factors V and VIII).

Multiple transfusions therefore lead to a coagulopathy. Most of the clotting factors are synthesised in the liver, although only factors II, VII, IX and X are dependent on vitamin K for their synthesis. In someone who is bleeding because of excessive warfarin administration, only fresh frozen plasma (FFP) will rapidly reverse the effect of warfarin. Vitamin K will act more slowly and, in addition, prevents re-anticoagulation with warfarin for up to a week.

1.34 Answer: C

The treatment of pulmonary embolism is i.v. heparin and warfarin in the longer term. Operations involving the knee, hip and pelvis are most commonly associated with DVT.

Regional anaesthesia on patients receiving prophylactic subcutaneous heparin is controversial. However, several large surveys have shown no increase in incidence of haematoma formation. HRT and low-oestrogen/progesterone oral contraceptives are not associated with an increased incidence of deep venous thrombosis.

1.35 Answers: A B C

The blood gases reveal hypoxia and respiratory alkalosis from hyperventilation: type 1 respiratory failure. This could be due to altitude. At sea level, barometric pressure is 100 kPa and air contains 21% oxygen. The partial pressure of oxygen being inspired is therefore 21 kPa. At 5500 metres, for example, the barometric pressure is about 50 kPa, so the partial pressure of oxygen being inspired is only about 10 kPa. The arterial oxygen tension might be expected, therefore, to be about 8 kPa. Hypoxic stimulation of the peripheral chemoreceptors causes hyperventilation and a respiratory alkalosis. A pneumothorax, if large enough, can cause hypoxia as blood passes through the non-ventilated lung causing a shunt. The hypoxia stimulates ventilation and the $PaCO_2$ is lowered. However, in most small spontaneous pneumothoraces, the blood gases are normal. In hysteria, there is hyperventilation and a resultant respiratory alkalosis, but the $PaCO_2$ will be normal. Salicylate poisoning initially causes hyperventilation and a respiratory alkalosis due to direct stimulation of the respiratory centre. In severe overdose, there is uncoupling of oxidative phosphorylation and a metabolic acidosis. Carbon monoxide (CO) has an affinity for oxygen 240 times that of haemoglobin. Thus, in CO poisoning, there is usually a reduced PaO_2 and compensatory hyperventilation.

1.36 Answers: A E

Acute hypovolaemia causes a release of catecholamines leading to tachycardia and vasoconstriction. The blood flow to essential organs such as kidneys and brain is preserved unless the hypovolaemia is severe. There is activation of the compensatory antidiuretic hormone (ADH) and renin–angiotensin–aldosterone systems leading to salt and water retention. The PaO_2 and $PaCO_2$ are generally unchanged.

There may be an increase in physiological dead space as areas of lung may be underperfused and, as a result, an increased alveolar-to-arterial oxygen gradient.

1.37 Answers: A B C D

Platelets are necessary for clot retraction to occur; clot retraction is caused by platelet contractile microfilaments. Contraction of the microfilaments is activated by calcium ions (released from stores in the mitochondria and endoplasmic reticulum) and thrombin (precursor prothrombin). In order to form a clot a platelet plug must be bound by fibrin which is formed by the action of thrombin on fibrinogen.

1.38 Answers: A B C D E

An increase in $PaCO_2$ leads to release of catecholamines from the adrenal medulla and the resulting sympathetic overactivity is manifested as tachycardia, hypertension, sweating and mydriasis.

Hypercarbia also causes narcosis and unconsciousness.

1.39 Answers: A B D E

A Valsalva manoeuvre is a forced expiration against a closed glottis.

This leads to a raised intrathoracic pressure. The initial effect is a transient increase in blood pressure as blood is squeezed out of the thorax and into the systemic circulation. There is then, however, a reduction in venous return to the right side of the heart, leading to a reduction in stroke volume, cardiac output and blood pressure.

The baroreceptor-mediated compensation causes a tachycardia and increased peripheral vascular resistance. Once the manoeuvre is terminated, the venous return is restored and the blood pressure rises transiently to a level greater than normal. A baroreceptor-mediated bradycardia occurs at this stage.

1.40 Answers: A D E

Albumin has a molecular weight of about 65,000 Da. It is synthesised in the liver, and is therefore reduced in liver disease.

Malabsorption leads to reduced absorption of the amino acids necessary for albumin synthesis. The normal serum albumin concentration is 35–50 g/l. Albumin exerts several effects including: maintenance of colloid osmotic pressure, free radical scavenging and binding and transport of drugs.

1.41 Answers: A E

The metabolic rate decreases during sleep and hypothermia. Tidal volume decreases with deepening levels of sleep. Respiratory rate increases slightly in all stages of sleep but the minute volume is progressively reduced in parallel with the tidal volume. The minute volume is increased by an increase in body acidity to create a compensatory respiratory alkalosis by removing carbon dioxide from the body.

At high altitude the decrease in inspired gas PO_2 reduces alveolar and therefore arterial PO_2. The actual decrease in alveolar PO_2 is tempered by hyperventilation caused by the hypoxic drive to ventilation.

1.42 Answers: A B C E

The oxyhaemoglobin dissociation curve is moved to the right (the Bohr effect) by an increase in temperature, hydrogen ion concentration (lowered pH, acidosis) and 2,3-diphosphoglycerate (2,3-DPG). Anaemia is associated with an increase in 2,3-DPG, and therefore a right shift of the curve. A shift of the curve to the right facilitates oxygen delivery to the tissues.

1.43 Answers: D E

Blood returning to the right side of the heart has an oxygen saturation of about 75%, the tissues having extracted about 25% of the oxygen delivered to them. Blood is then pumped through the pulmonary artery and is oxygenated as it passes through the lungs before returning to the left atrium via the pulmonary veins. The pressures in the heart are:

right atrium 5 mmHg
right ventricle 25/5 mmHg
pulmonary artery 25/10 mmHg
left atrium 8 mmHg
left ventricle 125/8 mmHg

1.44 Answer: C

The autonomic nervous system consists of sympathetic and parasympathetic systems. The neurotransmitter at all autonomic ganglia is acetylcholine (ACh). All pre-ganglionic fibres (sympathetic or parasympathetic) release ACh, including fibres which supply the chromaffin cells of the adrenal medulla. The neurotransmitter at the post-ganglionic nerve endings is ACh for the parasympathetic system and noradrenaline for the sympathetic system, except sympathetic fibres to sweat glands which produce ACh.

1.45 Answers: B D E

Sodium reabsorption in the kidney is mainly under the influence of the renin–angiotensin–aldosterone system. Renin is produced by the juxtaglomerular apparatus of the kidney in response to reduced blood flow or hyponatraemia. Renin circulates in the blood and acts on angiotensinogen, produced by the lungs, converting it to angiotensin. Angiotensin acts as a vasoconstrictor and stimulates production of aldosterone by the adrenal cortex. Aldosterone acts on the proximal tubules of the kidney to promote sodium reabsorption. Antidiuretic hormone (ADH) is produced by the posterior pituitary and acts on the collecting ducts to promote water reabsorption. The loop of Henle acts to produce a hypertonic renal medulla. This involves active chloride, but passive sodium reabsorption.

1.46 Answers: A B C D E

Block of the cervical sympathetic ganglia leads to Horner's syndrome, which is characterised by miosis, enophthalmos, anhidrosis, nasal congestion, ptosis and dilatation of conjunctival vessels.

1.47 Answers: A C D E

Metabolic acidosis is caused by (1) either ingestion or production of excess acid (eg salicylate poisoning or diabetic ketoacidosis) or (2) either failure to excrete acid or excessive loss of bicarbonate (eg renal failure or diarrhoea). Transplantation of the ureters into the colon causes a hyperchloraemic acidosis.

1.48 Answers: B C D E

Pyloric stenosis causes vomiting of acidic stomach contents (hydrogen and chloride ions) without loss of the alkaline small bowel contents. Thus, a metabolic alkalosis with hypochloraemia ensues. The body attempts to compensate for metabolic alkalosis by hypoventilation and by renal retention of hydrogen ions. However, vomiting also leads to hypovolaemia and dehydration and correction of this takes precedence over correction of acid–base status. Thus the kidney paradoxically produces potassium and acid urine by excreting hydrogen ions in exchange for sodium and water.

Thus the metabolic alkalosis is exacerbated and in addition hypokalaemia produced.

1.49 Answers: A B C E

Red blood cells contains a number of surface antigens. The ABO and Rhesus are two separate systems which are used to type red cells and avoid haemolytic transfusion reactions.

The following table shows how the ABO system works.

Blood group	Red cell antigens	Antibodies
A	A	Anti-B
B	B	Anti-A
AB	A + B	None
O	None	Anti-A/Anti-B

With the Rhesus system, a person who is Rhesus positive expresses the Rhesus antigen on red cells; a Rhesus-negative person has no Rhesus antigen on the red cells. A person who is blood group O Rhesus-negative thus has neither ABO nor Rhesus antigens and is a universal donor. Other less antigenic red cell surface antigens include Kell, Kidd and Duffy.

1.50 Answer: D

Intubation of the right main bronchus leads initially to elevated inflation pressure and hypoxaemia. At a later stage it may lead to collapse of the right upper lobe. There is no effect on the blood pressure nor is there hypercapnia.

1.51 Answers: All false

The normal arterial pH range is 7.35–7.45. A pH of 7.4 is equivalent to a hydrogen ion concentration of 40 nmol/l. With blood gas the measured parameters are PO_2, PCO_2 and pH. From these measurements, other parameters can be derived, eg bicarbonate, base excess, oxygen content and oxygen saturation.

The arterial pH is maintained within narrow limits mainly by excretion of CO_2 by the lungs and to a lesser extent by excretion of hydrogen ions by the kidney (the bicarbonate system). The neonatal pH range is lower than that of the adult.

1.52 Answer: B

The time taken for the depolarisation wave to pass from the sinoatrial node, across the atria and through the atrioventricular node into ventricular muscle is called the PR interval. The normal PR interval is 0.12–0.2 s. The QT interval represents the total time taken by ventricular depolarisation and repolarisation. It is normally <0.44 s. The QRS complex represents ventricular depolarisation and conduction delay is present when its duration is >0.12 s. The T wave represents ventricular repolarisation.

The ST interval is the transient period when no further electrical current can be passed through the myocardium.

1.53 Answers: B C D E

Dead space is the volume of inspired air that takes no part in gas exchange. It is made up of the volume of the conducting airways (anatomical dead space) and that part of the alveolar volume occupying alveoli which are inadequately perfused with blood and therefore not taking part in gas exchange (alveolar dead space).

Physiological dead space equals anatomical dead space plus alveolar dead space. The anatomical dead space may be measured using Fowler's method. It is the physiological dead space that is derived from the Bohr equation. The functional residual capacity (FRC) is the amount of gas remaining in the lungs at the end of a normal expiration (about 2.5 litres in an adult). It cannot be measured directly. It can be measured using the helium dilution method, or by a nitrogen washout technique or with a body plethysmograph.

1.54 Answers: B C E

The GFR is the volume of plasma (ml) filtered by the kidneys per minute. It is normally about 125 ml/min. GFR can be measured using the relationship GFR = UV/P (where U = urine concentration of substance, V = volume of urine produced per minute and P = concentration of substance in plasma) for any substance that is freely filtered and not reabsorbed or secreted. Inulin, a fructose polysaccharide, fulfils these criteria. Sodium reabsorption in the renal tubules leads to a low excretion rate and low urinary concentration of sodium.

1.55 Answers: A E

The basal metabolic rate (BMR) is the energy output per unit of time of an individual, determined at rest in a room at a comfortable temperature in the thermoneutral zone, 12–14 hours after the last meal. The BMR increases by 14% for every degree centigrade rise in body temperature. BMR is higher in males and children and decreases with age. Foods, especially protein, increase heat production by their 'specific dynamic action'. Most of this specific dynamic action is due to oxidative deamination of amino acids in the liver.

1.56 Answer: D

The best source of non-protein energy in parenteral nutrition is a balanced combination of carbohydrate and fat (usually 2/3 carbohydrate and 1/3 lipid). Glucose is the preferred intravenous carbohydrate source. It has been used in the past as the sole energy source but this has disadvantages: hyperglycaemia, fatty infiltration of the liver, excessive carbon dioxide production (requiring extra respiratory effort) and essential fatty acid deficiency. Nitrogen requirements are decreased in elderly, female, frail and starved patients. Factors which increase the nitrogen requirements are youth, male sex, large body frame, trauma and sepsis. The preferred choice of nitrogen for parenteral nutrition is a solution of L-amino acids. Glutamine is thought to play an important role in the maintenance of gut mucosal integrity.

1.57 Answers: A B E

The specific heat of blood and injectate is used in the calculations.

The Fick technique is used to measure cardiac output and blood flow to individual organs and is based on the Fick principle. This states that the amount of a substance taken up by an organ (or the body) per unit time is equal to the blood flow multiplied by the difference in concentration of that substance between arterial and mixed venous blood. In practice, the average steady-state oxygen consumption (VO_2) of the whole body is measured for about 15 minutes, during which time blood samples are taken from a systemic artery and pulmonary artery (mixed venous blood). The samples are then analysed for the oxygen content of arterial (C_aO_2) and mixed venous (C_vO_2) blood and cardiac output (Q) is calculated from:

$$Q \text{ (l/min)} = VO_2 \text{ (l/min)}/C_aO_2 - C_vO_2 \text{ (litre of } O_2 \text{ per litre of blood)}$$

The thermodilution technique involves injecting a solution that is colder than blood through the right atrial port of a pulmonary artery catheter and measuring the temperature change distally with a thermistor. Cardiac output is proportional to this temperature change divided by the area under the curve of temperature change against time. Pulmonary artery temperature variation occurs from right ventricle surface cooling from the overlying lung during panting, deep spontaneous respirations and with Valsalva manoeuvres.

1.58 Answers: A B D

The Glasgow Coma Scale consists of three categories with a score for each, totalled to give an overall score from 3 to 15.

Best motor response	Best verbal response	Eye opening
6 to command	5 fully orientated	4 spontaneous
5 localises to pain	4 confused	3 to command
4 withdrawal to pain	3 inappropriate words	2 to pain
3 flexes to pain	2 incomprehensible	1 none
2 extends to pain	sounds	
1 no response	1 no response	

As with central venous pressure (CVP) readings, changes in scores over time are often more useful than single values. There is a modified Glasgow Coma Scale for children which provides helpful information.

1.59 Answer: A

1 mmHg = 1.4 cmH$_2$O or 1 cmH$_2$O = 0.76 mmHg.

The CVP is a good indicator of right ventricular preload and right ventricular function. The CVP is a reasonable indicator of left atrial pressure in patients with normal myocardial and pulmonary function. The pulmonary artery catheter is a more reliable monitor for left-sided pressures and performance. Ideally the catheter tip should lie in the superior vena cava above the pericardial reflection to reduce the risk of thrombi, arrhythmias and cardiac tamponade if erosion and bleeding occur. The CVP primarily reflects right-sided function, therefore CVP can be normal in the presence of left ventricular failure and pulmonary oedema or raised in right-sided failure with normal left-sided function. Venoconstriction increases the CVP.

1.60 Answers: A E

Pulsatile veins may cause the pulse oximeters to under read as the technique cannot tell the difference between pulsating veins and arterioles, eg in tricuspid incompetence. The amount of transmitted light is sensed several hundred times per second to allow for precise estimation of the peak and trough of each pulse waveform. Pulse oximeters average their readings every 10–20 seconds so they cannot detect acute desaturation. They therefore give a comparatively late warning of, for example, failure of oxygen supply or oxygen failure. The light for measurement comes from light emitting diodes of wavelengths 660 nm and 940 nm.

For every 1% carboxyhaemoglobin circulating, the pulse oximeter over reads by about 1%: 50% of cigarette smokers have carboxyhaemoglobin levels of > 6%. Methaemoglobinaemia leads to a falsely low saturation. Other factors affecting the accuracy of pulse oximetry are methylene blue, indocyanine green, opaque nail varnish, extraneous light sources, peripheral vasoconstriction, excessive movement and drugs responsible for the production of methaemoglobinaemia, eg EDTA, local anaesthetic agents.

1.61 Answers: A C D

The stoichiometric concentration of a fuel and oxidising agent is the concentration at which all the combustible vapour and agent are completely used. Therefore the most violent and fastest reactions occur in stoichiometric mixtures. The risk of explosion is greater at stoichiometric concentrations. Nitrous oxide supports combustion more fiercely than oxygen. Nitrous oxide breaks down to oxygen and nitrogen with heat and produces further energy; thus reactions may be more vigorous with nitrous oxide than with oxygen alone.

1 microjoule of energy is sufficient for reactions in oxygen while 100 microjoules is required with air. The risk of sparking is greater in cold, dry environments.

1.62 Answers: B C

The post-tetanic count is useful during periods of intense neuromuscular blockade (when there is no response to train of four stimulation). A 50-Hz tetanic stimulus is applied for 5 seconds followed by a pause of 3 seconds; then the number of twitches produced by single pulses at 1 Hz is counted. If the count is 6 then the first reaction to a train of four will occur in less than 10 minutes; if the count is only 2, the response will require 15 minutes or longer.

Train of four stimulation consists of 4 supramaximal stimuli at 2 Hz.

If large amounts of suxamethonium are used, dual block, in which features of a non-depolarising neuromuscular block gradually replace those of depolarising blockade, may supervene.

Use of the orbicularis oculi (facial nerve) underestimates the degree of neuromuscular blockade because of direct muscle stimulation and relative insensitivity of the facial muscles to neuromuscular blockers. This is in contrast to using abductor pollicis (ulnar nerve) which is more sensitive than the diaphragm and vocal cords to neuromuscular blockers.

1.63 Answers: A B C E

A sine wave pattern is used for cutting and a damped or pulsed sine wave pattern for coagulation. In bipolar diathermy the current passes from one blade of a pair of forceps to the other, ie passes across the tissue held between the tips of a pair of forceps. The circuit is earth-free – no plate electrode is required. The current does not pass through any part of the patient's body other than that between the forceps. The power required is small and it is electrically safer than unipolar diathermy. However, it is only suitable for the coagulation of small pieces of tissues or blood vessels, eg in ophthalmic surgery or neurosurgery.

1.64 Answer: C

Maintaining an ambient temperature of 22°C to 24°C and a humidity of 50%–70% minimises heat loss. Giving cold fluids into a central vein decreases core temperature more rapidly than giving them peripherally. Phenothiazines have an alpha-adrenoceptor antagonist effect and therefore cause vasodilatation. Space blankets are made of shiny, reflective, metallised plastic foil and should not be used in theatre because of the increased risks of burns and electrical shock, and because they are made of highly flammable material.

1.65 Answers: B E

The width of the cuff should be 20% greater than the diameter of the arm. Too narrow a cuff leads to falsely high blood pressure readings whereas too loose a cuff produces falsely low pressures. For accurate measurement of blood pressure, there should be a fast cuff inflation to avoid venous congestion and a slow deflation to allow enough time to detect the arterial pulsation. If the cuff pressure is released too quickly the pressure recorded tends to be erroneously low because of the delay between passing the real pressure and seeing the reading. The resistance to occlusion of the blood vessel wall by the cuff is increased in atherosclerosis.

1.66 Answer: D

The saturated vapour pressure (SVP) is not linearly related to temperature; it increases with temperature according to a complex equation which approximates to an exponential relation. When SVP equals atmospheric pressure, the liquid boils. SVP depends on the temperature and the nature of the liquid only. The SVP for water at body temperature is 6.3 kPa.

1.67 Answers: B D

Flow rate is described by the Hagen–Poiseuille equation:

$V = (\Delta P \pi r^4)/8\mu$

Where V = rate of flow, P = pressure gradient along the tube, r = radius of the tube, μ = viscosity of fluid and l = length of the tube.

1.68 Answer: D

The problem of nitrogen narcosis can be avoided by breathing a helium/oxygen mixture rather than a nitrogen/oxygen mixture because helium is only half as soluble as nitrogen so that less is dissolved in the tissues. Helium is less dense than nitrogen, which decreases gas flow resistance and therefore the work of breathing.

Helium/oxygen mixtures have a greater viscosity than nitrogen/oxygen mixtures. This is why helium is of no use in lower airway obstruction (eg asthma) where flow is laminar and therefore depends on viscosity rather than density.

1.69 Answers: A B C

End-inspiratory and end-expiratory values for CVP in healthy individuals are normally –5 and –3 cmH₂O, respectively. Right atrial pressures do not always reflect left atrial pressures, eg left ventricular failure or infarction, valvular heart disease.

1.70 Answers: C D E

Soda lime contains 80% calcium hydroxide, 4% sodium hydroxide, 14%–20% added water content and a pH indicator. The sodium hydroxide improves the reactivity of the mixture and has hygroscopic properties (binding the necessary added water in the mixture). The addition of silica to help form the required granule size is no longer needed in modern manufacturing processes.

Potassium hydroxide, which was thought to improve the activity of soda lime when cold, is no longer added. The reaction of carbon dioxide with soda lime is an exothermic reaction; the temperature within the canister can reach 60°C.

1.71 Answers: C D E

At 4°C, bacterial replication in blood is inhibited. An increase in temperature, acidosis, raised carbon dioxide level and increased 2,3-diphosphoglycerate levels shift the O_2 dissociation curve to the right. Rapid transfusion of cold blood can cause cardiac arrest; cold blood is arrhythmogenic.

1.72 Answers: A B C D E

The relative humidity in theatre should be 50%–70%. This is a compromise. Too high a humidity is uncomfortable and tiring for the staff but a low humidity increases the risk of explosion due to static electricity. Air contains approximately 79% nitrogen and nitrogen does not support combustion. An explosive mixture with air requires about 100 microjoules of energy to ignite it; this is 100 times the energy required to ignite an explosive mixture with oxygen.

An area extending for 25 cm around any part of the anaesthetic circuit or gas paths of an anaesthetic apparatus should be regarded as a zone of risk (AAGBI 1971). It is the area of theatre where mixtures of anaesthetic agents may be explosive. Within the zone of risk there should be no naked flames, all electrical switches should be spark proof and all parts should be made of conductive (antistatic) materials. Antistatic rubber containing carbon has enough conductivity to remove static electricity, but sufficient resistance to prevent a spark occurring from too rapid a discharge.

The floor is constructed of terrazzo screed which acts as a large capacitor. The resistance of the floor over a distance of 60 cm should be 20,000–5,000,000 Ω. This allows the slow discharge of current to earth. Wool and nylon readily acquire static charge.

1.73 Answers: A C

The critical temperature is the temperature above which a substance cannot be liquefied no matter how much pressure is applied. A vapour is a substance in the gaseous phase below its critical temperature, ie its constituent particles may enter the liquid form. Strictly speaking a substance is a gas when at a temperature above its critical temperature. The critical temperature of oxygen is –118 °C.

1.74 Answer: E

Nitrous oxide is stored at a pressure of 44 bar (4400 kPa) as a liquid in equilibrium with its vapour. Entonox is stored at a pressure of 137 bar (13,700 kPa) as a gas. A full cylinder of oxygen is stored at 137 bar (13,700 kPa). Medical gases are supplied as dry gases to prevent corrosion, condensation and frost in cylinders, pipes or valves.

Entonox should not be stored below its pseudocritical temperature of –6°C, the temperature at which it may separate out into its constituent parts (lamination).

1.75 Answers: B C D

Force is measured in newtons. Pressure is the force applied or distributed over a surface, ie force per unit area. The SI unit of pressure is the pascal and 1 pascal is a pressure of 1 newton active over an area of 1 square metre (1 Pa = 1 N/m^2). Cylinders are normally calibrated in gauge pressure, ie the pressure above atmospheric pressure. Absolute pressure = gauge pressure + atmospheric pressure (= 137 bar + 1 bar = 138 bar in the case of oxygen cylinders). The reading will be increased in the case of a water manometer and decreased in the case of a mercury manometer due to the effect of surface tension.

1.76 Answers: All false

Turbulent flow is directly proportional to both the radius of the orifice squared and the square root of pressure and inversely proportional to the square root of the density of the fluid.

Reynolds' number = density × velocity × diameter of tube/ viscosity. If Reynolds' number exceeds 2000, turbulent flow is more likely. Warming gases decreases their density and increases their viscosity, thereby decreasing Reynolds' number and making turbulent flow less likely. Turbulent flow is more likely in the trachea. In the bronchial tree, flow is mainly transitional and true laminar flow probably only occurs in the very small airways.

1.77 Answers: B C

Boyle's Law: at constant temperature, the volume of a given mass of gas varies inversely with the absolute pressure.

Charles' Law: at constant pressure, the volume of a given mass of gas varies directly with the absolute temperature.

Third Gas Law: at constant volume, the absolute pressure of a given mass of gas varies directly with temperature.

Dalton's Law of Partial Pressures: in a mixture of gases the pressure exerted by each gas is the same as that which it would exert if it alone occupied the container.

Alteration of the state of a gas without allowing the temperature to alter is known as adiabatic change.

1.78 Answers: B C D

The critical temperature is the temperature above which a substance cannot be liquefied by pressure alone. The critical temperature applies to a single gas. The pseudocritical temperature is the temperature at which gas mixtures separate out into their constituent parts.

1.79 Answers: B E

Absolute humidity is the amount of water vapour per unit volume of gas at a given temperature and pressure. In the upper trachea absolute humidity is 34 g/m³ or 34 mg/l. Humidification avoids the need for latent heat of vaporisation which normally accounts for 15% of total heat loss within the trachea. Less than 2% of basal heat loss is used to warm the gases. HMEs are now > 70% efficient and can give a humidity of the inspired gases of >20 g/m³. Each HME should only be used for a maximum of 24 hours. There is a risk of increased airways resistance (ie increased work of breathing) due to dry crusted secretions and infection.

1.80 Answers: A B C D

Thermocouples rely on the Seebeck effect, ie when two dissimilar conductors are joined together to form a circuit, a potential difference is generated, the size of which is proportional to the difference in temperature between the two junctions. In order to measure temperature one junction has to be kept at a constant temperature.

Alcohol thermometers are more suitable for measuring very low temperatures as mercury solidifies at –39°C. However, they are unsuitable for measuring high temperatures as alcohol boils at 78.5°C.

The resistance thermometer relies on the fact that the electrical resistance of a metal increases linearly with temperature. A thermistor also uses resistance to measure temperature. It consists of a bead of metal oxide, the resistance of which falls exponentially as temperature rises. The interferometer is used for gas analysis.

1.81 Answers: A D

The Wright's respirometer is a turbine flowmeter used to measure expiratory gas volumes. It gives falsely low readings when the ventilation volumes to be measured are small and when the vanes are wet. It over reads when flow rates or tidal volumes are great. It also gives slightly higher readings with mixtures of nitrous oxide and oxygen than for air. To improve accuracy, the respirometer should be positioned as close as possible to the patient's trachea on the expiratory limb of the breathing circuit. The Wright's respirometer is calibrated for use for tidal volume measurement and for tidal ventilation. Its calibration is inaccurate if it is used to measure a continuous flow.

1.82 Answers: A C D

Evoked potentials (EPs) are electrical potentials recorded from the central nervous system or peripherally following repetitive central or peripheral stimulation. EPs can be sensory (eg somatosensory, auditory or visual) or motor.

1.83 Answers: C D

The half-life is the time taken for the initial response to fall to half its value. As an alternative to half-life, the rate of an exponential process can be measured by its time constant. It is equal to the time at which the process would have been complete had the initial rate of change continued. After 1 time constant the process is 63% complete, after 2 time constants it is 86.5% complete, after 3 time constants it is 95% complete and after 4 time constants it is 99.75% complete.

1.84 Answers: A C D E

Resistance = driving pressure/gas flow rate. Driving pressure is the difference between alveolar and mouth pressures and can be measured with the body plethysmograph. Gas flow rate can be measured with a pneumotachograph. Airway resistance is the pressure difference between the alveoli and the mouth per unit of air flow. It is therefore measured in $cmH_2O/l/per$ s or $kPa/l/per$ s.

Airway resistance increases during inhalational anaesthesia. This may be caused by the reduced functional residual capacity and lung volume or by the tubes and connections of the breathing system.

Positive end-expiration pressure (PEEP) reduces airway resistance according to the inverse relationship between lung volume and airway resistance; it recruits previously closed alveoli.

1.85 Answers: A B C E

Microshock refers to the application of a small current close to or directly to the heart. Cardiac pacing wires and invasive monitoring catheters provide a conductive route to the endothelium of the heart. Blood and saline can act as electrical conductors. Under these circumstances currents as low as 100 µA can result in ventricular fibrillation. Ideally two or more pieces of earthed equipment should be at the same potential to avoid leakage currents which can give rise to microelectrocution. However, it is virtually impossible to ensure that all earth connections which are made to the patient, either deliberately or accidentally, are at the same potential. It is therefore recommended that patients are isolated from earth by using isolated or floating circuits.

1.86 Answers: A C

Refer to Answer 1.57.

1.87 Answers: A B C D

The Lack system is a coaxial modification of the Magill Mapleson A system. The Magill and Lack systems are efficient for spontaneous ventilation; fresh gas flow (FGF) required = alveolar minute ventilation (approximately 70 ml/kg). However, although they can be used for controlled ventilation, they are very inefficient; FGF required = 3 × alveolar minute ventilation.

1.88 Answers: A B C D

The central venous pressure (CVP) is expressed as cmH_2O or mmHg above a point level with the right atrium, eg midaxillary line. When changing the position of the patient it is important that the pressure recorded always be related to the level of the right atrium.

Misplacement of the catheter may lead to inaccuracies, eg if the catheter tip is in the right ventricle; this leads to an unexpectedly high pressure with pronounced oscillations. This is easily distinguished when the waveform is displayed. The upper end of the manometer column is open to air via a cotton wool filter. The filter must stay dry to maintain direct connection with the atmosphere.

Straining causes a raised intrathoracic pressure, increasing CVP.

Measurement of the CVP is useful in shock and hypovolaemia.

1.89 Answers: A B C D E

Static electricity and dirt on the bobbin can both cause the bobbin to stick. Dirt is a particular problem at low flow rates when the clearance between the bobbin and flowmeter wall is narrow. Each rotameter is calibrated for a specific gas at room temperature and pressure. Minute volume divider ventilators exert back pressure as they cycle. A flow restrictor can be fitted downstream of the flowmeters to prevent this from happening. As altitude increases barometric pressure decreases. At low flow rates, flow is laminar and dependent on gas viscosity, a property which is independent of altitude. At high flow rates, flow becomes turbulent and is dependent on density, a property which is influenced by altitude.

The decrease in density at altitude increases the actual flow rate and so the flowmeter under reads.

1.90 Answers: B E

Capnography works on the absorption of infra-red light by carbon dioxide (CO_2). Collision broadening is where the absorption of carbon dioxide is increased due to the presence of nitrous oxide. This occurs because carbon dioxide can transfer some of its absorbed infra-red energy to nitrous oxide molecules when they collide. This results in the CO_2 molecules being able to absorb more energy than would otherwise be the case. The absorption spectrum of the nitrous oxide is broadened and hence the term 'collision broadening'. The P_aCO_2/P_eCO_2 gradient in normal subjects is approximately 0.4–0.7 kPa. The difference increases in V/Q mismatch.

Multiple Choice Question Paper 2

90 Questions: time allowed 3 hours.

Indicate your answers with a tick or cross in the spaces provided.

2.1 **Recognised complications of dextran infusions are**

- A antigenic reactions
- B problems with cross matching of blood
- C an increase in venous thrombosis
- D renal failure
- E an increase in rouleaux formation

2.2 **The level of serum potassium may be**

- A increased by suxamethonium
- B increased by thiopentone
- C increased by metabolic alkalosis
- D affected by extensive burns
- E reduced by D-tubocurarine

2.3 **Non-depolarising muscle relaxants**

- A produce post-tetanic facilitation
- B all have their action prolonged by alkalosis
- C produce fasciculation
- D can exhibit dual block
- E have a prolonged action in severe hypothermia

2.4 **Convulsions occurring intra-operatively or in the early postoperative period may be due to**

- A ether
- B suxamethonium
- C isoflurane
- D bupivacaine
- E hypoxia

2.5 After intravenous thiopentone, the following may occur

- ❏ A severe hypotension
- ❏ B respiratory depression
- ❏ C liver toxicity
- ❏ D pain at the injection site
- ❏ E epileptic convulsions

2.6 At equivalent minimum alveolar concentration (MAC), comparing halothane with enflurane

- ❏ A enflurane causes more respiratory depression than halothane
- ❏ B enflurane causes more cardiac arrhythmias than halothane
- ❏ C enflurane causes a greater fall in cardiac output than halothane
- ❏ D both release inorganic fluoride ions
- ❏ E enflurane has a higher boiling point than halothane

2.7 Digoxin is indicated in

- ❏ A atrial flutter
- ❏ B 2:1 block
- ❏ C ventricular tachycardia
- ❏ D nodal tachycardia
- ❏ E Stokes-Adams attacks

2.8 Propranolol is contraindicated in

- ❏ A bronchial asthma
- ❏ B the presence of a low serum potassium
- ❏ C paroxysmal nocturnal dyspnoea
- ❏ D patients already on digoxin
- ❏ E atrial fibrillation

2.9 Dopamine infused at a dosage of 10 µg/kg per min may produce

- ❏ A increased urinary output
- ❏ B increased sodium output
- ❏ C increased cardiac output
- ❏ D multiple ventricular extrasystoles
- ❏ E an unchanged peripheral resistance

2.10 Regarding ketamine

- ❏ A   intracranial pressure is raised
- ❏ B   it causes muscle relaxation
- ❏ C   it relaxes the uterus
- ❏ D   it is excreted in the urine
- ❏ E   premedication with atropine is advisable when it is used

2.11 Sodium dantrolene

- ❏ A   is a neuromuscular blocker
- ❏ B   may cause a dangerous rise in the serum calcium
- ❏ C   can be used preoperatively to reduce suxamethonium pains
- ❏ D   is useful in the treatment of malignant hyperpyrexia
- ❏ E   is a skeletal muscle relaxant

2.12 Isoflurane

- ❏ A   has the same molecular weight as enflurane
- ❏ B   if put in a calibrated halothane vaporiser (ie Fluotec), a dangerously high concentration of isoflurane will be delivered
- ❏ C   reduces the blood pressure, mainly by depressing cardiac output
- ❏ D   has a MAC of 1.68%
- ❏ E   causes minimal changes in cerebral blood flow at light levels of anaesthesia

2.13 Morphine

- ❏ A   may cause histamine release
- ❏ B   decreases catecholamine levels
- ❏ C   causes miosis
- ❏ D   causes vomiting by direct stimulation of the vomiting centre
- ❏ E   causes markedly raised arterial PCO_2 with normal therapeutic dosage

2.14 Chlorpromazine

- ❏ A   is a weak antihistamine
- ❏ B   is an α-blocker
- ❏ C   can cause Parkinsonism
- ❏ D   is an anti-emetic
- ❏ E   has an atropine-like action

2.15 Chlorpropamide

- ❏ A has a half-life of 12 hours
- ❏ B is mainly metabolised in the liver
- ❏ C causes alcohol intolerance in about 30% of patients
- ❏ D acts by stimulating insulin production
- ❏ E results in unwanted effects twice as commonly as tolbutamide

2.16 The MAC value of an inhalational anaesthetic agent will be influenced by

- ❏ A the age of the patient
- ❏ B the concomitant administration of morphine
- ❏ C a change in the arterial PCO_2 from 3.5 to 6.5 kPa
- ❏ D its blood/gas partition coefficient
- ❏ E the use of nitrous oxide with it

2.17 Halothane decreases the blood pressure as a result of

- ❏ A direct myocardial depression
- ❏ B peripheral vasodilatation
- ❏ C a central action on the vasomotor centre
- ❏ D ganglion blockade
- ❏ E baroreceptor inhibition

2.18 Bupivacaine

- ❏ A produces depolarisation in the neural membrane of peripheral nerves
- ❏ B is detoxified in the liver
- ❏ C is an ester
- ❏ D can cause methaemoglobinaemia
- ❏ E recommended dose in a 75-kg man is 30 ml of 0.5%

2.19 The following are anticonvulsant

- ❏ A diazepam
- ❏ B chlormethiazole
- ❏ C oxazepam
- ❏ D chlorpropamide
- ❏ E thiopentone

2.20 Albumin

- ❏ A has a molecule weight of approximately 65,000 Daltons
- ❏ B is increased in chronic liver disease
- ❏ C is increased in malabsorption syndrome
- ❏ D makes a significant contribution to plasma oncotic pressure
- ❏ E has a normal value of 34–45 g/l

2.21 The following cause methaemoglobinaemia

- ❏ A atropine
- ❏ B prilocaine
- ❏ C methylene blue
- ❏ D cyanide
- ❏ E higher oxides of nitrogen

2.22 The following are anti-emetics

- ❏ A hyoscine
- ❏ B carbimazole
- ❏ C perphenazine
- ❏ D apomorphine
- ❏ E cyclizine

2.23 Thiazide diuretics

- ❏ A act on the proximal convoluted tubule
- ❏ B cause hyponatraemia
- ❏ C increase serum uric acid
- ❏ D cause hypercalcaemia
- ❏ E potentiate digoxin

2.24 Ketamine causes

- ❏ A bradycardia
- ❏ B postural hypotension
- ❏ C increased intracranial pressure
- ❏ D delirium
- ❏ E muscle rigidity

2.25 The following potentiate a competitive neuromuscular block

- ❏ A   increased serum magnesium
- ❏ B   increased serum calcium
- ❏ C   decreased serum potassium
- ❏ D   hyperventilation
- ❏ E   increased or decreased pH

2.26 Sodium nitroprusside cyanide toxicity is

- ❏ A   due to free cyanide
- ❏ B   due to thiocyanate
- ❏ C   worse in the presence of vitamin B12 deficiency
- ❏ D   worse in liver rhodanese deficiency
- ❏ E   dose-dependent

2.27 Propranolol

- ❏ A   can cause hypoglycaemia
- ❏ B   causes bradycardia
- ❏ C   is a bronchoconstrictor
- ❏ D   acts via cyclic AMP
- ❏ E   is potentiated by enoximone

2.28 Frusemide

- ❏ A   can cause a reduction in blood sugar
- ❏ B   decreases blood volume
- ❏ C   reduces osmolality in the renal tubules
- ❏ D   acts in the proximal convoluted tubule
- ❏ E   causes hyperkalaemia

2.29 Ventricular tachycardia can be abolished by

- ❏ A   digoxin
- ❏ B   lignocaine
- ❏ C   verapamil
- ❏ D   disopyramide
- ❏ E   adenosine

2.30 The speed of induction of an inhalational agent is increased by

- ❏ A hypovolaemia
- ❏ B hyperventilation
- ❏ C increased cardiac output
- ❏ D high solubility of the agent
- ❏ E polycythaemia

2.31 Long-term deficiency of adrenal cortical hormones causes

- ❏ A hyperpigmentation
- ❏ B hypovolaemia
- ❏ C hyponatraemia
- ❏ D hypokalaemia
- ❏ E decrease in anterior pituitary functions

2.32 Angiotensin II

- ❏ A stimulates the thirst centre
- ❏ B causes marked arteriolar vasoconstriction
- ❏ C causes venoconstriction
- ❏ D causes release of aldosterone from the zona glomerulosa
- ❏ E is metabolised in the lungs

2.33 Gastrin is

- ❏ A released in response to acid in the antrum
- ❏ B released in response to ethanol in the antrum
- ❏ C released from the fundus
- ❏ D increased by acetylcholine
- ❏ E increased by sympathetic stimulation

2.34 Clearance

- ❏ A equals renal excretion divided by plasma concentration
- ❏ B of urea equals GFR
- ❏ C of PAH equals renal plasma blood flow
- ❏ D of inulin is less than that of glucose
- ❏ E of free water is greater than that of inulin

2.35 Physiological dead space

- [ ] A changes with posture
- [ ] B decreases with exercise
- [ ] C includes anatomical dead space
- [ ] D is responsible for the difference between mixed expired gas and alveolar gas
- [ ] E is diffusion dependent

2.36 Lung surfactant

- [ ] A decreases compliance
- [ ] B increases surface tension
- [ ] C is released from the pulmonary circulation
- [ ] D is made of molecules that are partly lipophilic and partly hydrophilic
- [ ] E is produced in type I pneumocytes

2.37 The pyramidal tract

- [ ] A is named after the cells in the cortex where it originates
- [ ] B has 1 million fibres, 80%–90% of which decussate in the medulla
- [ ] C comes from area IV of the cortex
- [ ] D is concerned with fine movements
- [ ] E will degenerate after decortication

2.38 Smooth, cardiac and skeletal muscle have the following in common

- [ ] A gap junctions where electrical transmission spreads from cell to cell
- [ ] B resting membrane potential of −90 mV
- [ ] C action potential duration 200 ms
- [ ] D all calcium ions for contraction come from intracellular storage
- [ ] E contraction depends on interaction between actin and myosin

2.39 Regarding the pulmonary circulation

☐ A   it contains 30% of the blood volume
☐ B   pulmonary vascular resistance increases with hypoxia
☐ C   pulmonary vascular resistance is markedly less than systemic vascular resistance
☐ D   pulmonary artery pressure is 25/9 mmHg
☐ E   pulmonary artery pressure increases with exercise

2.40 At birth

☐ A   the ductus arteriosus opens
☐ B   left atrial pressure decreases
☐ C   pulmonary vascular resistance increases
☐ D   intrapleural pressure rises
☐ E   fetal haemoglobin is immediately replaced by HbA

2.41 Carbon dioxide

☐ A   is mainly carried as carbamino compounds
☐ B   10%–15% is dissolved in the plasma
☐ C   crosses the placenta more easily than oxygen
☐ D   carriage in fetal haemoglobin is facilitated by deoxygenation
☐ E   is more soluble in blood than oxygen

2.42 In a fit young person, tachycardia will be seen with

☐ A   emotional syncope
☐ B   expiration
☐ C   decrease in blood pressure
☐ D   noradrenaline infusion
☐ E   increased circulating thyroxine

2.43 Hypoxaemia stimulates ventilation by an effect on

☐ A   the carotid body
☐ B   the carotid sinus
☐ C   central chemoreceptors in the medulla
☐ D   central respiratory neurones
☐ E   cortical cells

2.44 Concerning skeletal muscle

- [ ] A each fibre has one motor endplate
- [ ] B the motor endplate is at the proximal end of the fibre
- [ ] C depolarisation causes electrical changes only in the muscle fibre near the endplate
- [ ] D the resting potential difference at the endplate is 20 mV less than over the rest of the muscle
- [ ] E each fibre is no longer than 1 mm

2.45 Section of the dorsal root nerves C3–L2 causes

- [ ] A hypotonia
- [ ] B paralysis
- [ ] C loss of reflexes
- [ ] D loss of sensation
- [ ] E loss of supply to sympathetic sweat glands

2.46 In normal blood

- [ ] A 20 ml of oxygen is carried per 100 ml of plasma
- [ ] B oxygen combines with globin in haemoglobin
- [ ] C viscosity is largely due to red cells
- [ ] D as velocity increases, red cells accumulate in the centre of vessels
- [ ] E red cells metabolise glucose

2.47 Receptors in the carotid body

- [ ] A respond to increases in P_aCO_2 by increasing ventilation
- [ ] B respond to stagnant hypoxia
- [ ] C respond to haemorrhagic hypoxia
- [ ] D have the same blood flow (weight for weight) as the myocardium
- [ ] E do not respond to increasing pH by increasing ventilation

2.48 Valsalva manoeuvre is associated with

- [ ] A increased central venous pressure
- [ ] B decreased peripheral resistance
- [ ] C tachycardia
- [ ] D drop in blood pressure
- [ ] E increased blood volume in the pulmonary circulation

2.49 The cerebrospinal fluid

☐ A contains virtually no glucose
☐ B pH does not accurately reflect the plasma pH
☐ C is secreted by the choroid plexus
☐ D is reabsorbed by the arachnoid villi
☐ E pressure increases with compression of jugular veins

2.50 Agglutination will occur if the following donor blood is given to the following recipients

		Donor	Recipient
☐	A	Group O	Group AB
☐	B	Group A	Group O
☐	C	Group AB	Group A
☐	D	Group A	Group AB
☐	E	Group O	Group A

2.51 Concerning the transmitter at motor nerve terminals

☐ A it is formed from choline and acetyl coenzyme A
☐ B formation occurs in the cleft
☐ C it is broken down by pseudocholinesterase
☐ D it has a muscarinic action
☐ E release is increased by botulinum toxin

2.52 Enkephalin

☐ A is a pentapeptide
☐ B is the same as endorphin
☐ C has a long half-life in the brain
☐ D is mainly found in the pituitary
☐ E is an agonist at opiate receptors but is not antagonised by naloxone

2.53 The following are beta actions of adrenaline

- ❏ A pupil dilation
- ❏ B fine tremor
- ❏ C tachycardia
- ❏ D increase in cyclic AMP
- ❏ E vasoconstriction

2.54 The following are effects of cortisol

- ❏ A protein anabolism
- ❏ B osteoporosis
- ❏ C potassium retention
- ❏ D depression of function of the anterior pituitary
- ❏ E salt and water retention

2.55 The plasma osmolality decreases after infusion of

- ❏ A isotonic saline solution
- ❏ B vasopressin
- ❏ C aldosterone
- ❏ D isotonic glucose
- ❏ E 20% albumin solution

2.56 Thyroid stimulating hormone (TSH) produces

- ❏ A increased thyroidal uptake of iodine
- ❏ B increased coupling of monoiodotyrosine and diiodotyrosine
- ❏ C increased synthesis of thyroglobulin
- ❏ D increased cyclic AMP levels in thyroid cells
- ❏ E an increase in basal metabolic rate

2.57 Which of the following are not seen following total pancreatectomy?

- ❏ A little change in plasma insulin level
- ❏ B little change in plasma glucagon level
- ❏ C steatorrhoea
- ❏ D increased plasma levels of free fatty acids
- ❏ E decreased plasma P_aCO_2

2.58 Large doses of glucagon

- ❏ A increase the force of contraction of the myocardium
- ❏ B increase the concentration of amino acids in the plasma
- ❏ C increase the concentration of free fatty acids in the plasma
- ❏ D decrease the plasma sodium concentration
- ❏ E stimulate the sympathetic nervous system

2.59 A decreased extracellular fluid volume would be expected to cause an increased secretion of

- ❏ A vasopressin
- ❏ B renin
- ❏ C ACTH
- ❏ D thyroxine
- ❏ E progesterone

2.60 A high plasma calcium level causes

- ❏ A bone demineralisation
- ❏ B decreased secretion of calcitonin
- ❏ C increased formation of 1,25-dihydroxycholecalciferol
- ❏ D decreased blood coagulability
- ❏ E increased formation of 24,25-dihydroxycholecalciferol

2.61 A Wright's respirometer will give a reading that is lower than the actual value where there is

- ❏ A low flow of gas
- ❏ B 30% oxygen in the gas
- ❏ C nitrous oxide present
- ❏ D humidity in the respirometer
- ❏ E an intermittent flow of gas

2.62 Evoked potential techniques for measuring depth of anaesthesia utilise the following stimuli

- ❏ A auditory
- ❏ B oesophageal contractions
- ❏ C somatosensory
- ❏ D visual
- ❏ E magnetic resonance

2.63 Blood pressure measurements read 'high' when

- ❏ A there is a narrow cuff
- ❏ B the cuff is deflated slowly
- ❏ C the arm is held horizontal when the patient is sitting upright
- ❏ D the arm is obese
- ❏ E the arm muscles are held tight

2.64 Helium is used by divers because it

- ❏ A has a low viscosity
- ❏ B has no narcotic effect
- ❏ C diffuses easily through the nose
- ❏ D is more dense than air
- ❏ E can be liquefied

2.65 The chances of microshock occurring increases due to

- ❏ A saline-filled catheters
- ❏ B earth loop
- ❏ C multiple earth connections
- ❏ D isolated circuit
- ❏ E oesophageal electrocardiogram

2.66 The following are required to measure the cardiac output by the Fick principle

- ❏ A arterial oxygen content
- ❏ B venous oxygen content
- ❏ C oxygen uptake
- ❏ D respiratory quotient
- ❏ E arterial carbon monoxide content

2.67 The following apply to medical gases

❏ A the oxygen concentrator has air passed under pressure through a column of zeolite

❏ B nitrogen is a constituent of nitrous oxide in the concentration of 0.5%

❏ C helium is obtained by fractional distillation of atmospheric air

❏ D the main source of carbon dioxide gas is as the by-product of petroleum hydrocarbon reformation

❏ E nitrous oxide is manufactured by thermal decomposition of ammonium nitrate

2.68 In exponential change

❏ A the time constant is the time taken for the initial response to fall to half its value

❏ B in one time constant, 37% change is complete

❏ C in three time constants, 95% change is complete

❏ D the rate of change of a variable is proportional to the magnitude of the variable

❏ E the half-life is half the time constant

2.69 Airway resistance

❏ A can be measured by plethysmography

❏ B is measured in kPa per litre per second

❏ C increases during inhalational anaesthesia

❏ D increases at high inspiratory flow rates

❏ E decreases with the application of positive end-expiratory pressure

2.70 The single-breath nitrogen test measures

❏ A anatomical dead space

❏ B physiological dead space

❏ C distribution of gases

❏ D diffusing capacity

❏ E closing volume

2.71 The alveolar-to-arterial oxygen tension is increased from normal

- ☐ A with high inspired oxygen
- ☐ B during nitrous oxide uptake
- ☐ C in Fallot's tetralogy
- ☐ D with a decrease in functional residual capacity
- ☐ E in the elderly

2.72 With medical oxygen

- ☐ A the critical temperature is 36.5°C
- ☐ B manufacture is by the fractional distillation of air
- ☐ C explosions can occur if, under pressure, it comes into contact with oil or grease
- ☐ D convulsions can be caused if it is given under hyperbaric conditions
- ☐ E bone marrow depression can occur with prolonged administration

2.73 In nitrous oxide cylinders for medical use

- ☐ A the cylinder is initially full of liquid
- ☐ B nitrous oxide is produced by heating ammonium nitrate
- ☐ C contaminants may be tested for with moistened starch-iodide paper
- ☐ D the pressure gauge reading is proportional to the amount of nitrous oxide in the cylinder
- ☐ E contamination with nitric oxide may occur

2.74 Soda lime

- ☐ A is mainly calcium carbonate
- ☐ B can be used to scavenge nitrous oxide
- ☐ C needs water to absorb carbon dioxide
- ☐ D in a properly packed canister, half the volume should be space between the granules
- ☐ E gets hot in use

2.75 Regarding the Magill circuit

- ❏ A   it is an example of a Mapleson A circuit
- ❏ B   it is functionally similar to the Lack circuit
- ❏ C   it is suitable for children over 25 kg
- ❏ D   it is efficient during IPPV
- ❏ E   during spontaneous ventilation, rebreathing and hypercarbia will occur if the fresh gas flow is less than the minute volume

2.76 Inaccuracies in the measurement of central venous pressure may arise from

- ❏ A   a change in the position of the patient
- ❏ B   misplacement of the catheter
- ❏ C   wetting of the cotton wool plug in the top of the manometer tube
- ❏ D   straining during respiration
- ❏ E   arterial hypotension

2.77 The accuracy of a rotameter may be affected by

- ❏ A   dirt on the bobbin
- ❏ B   static electricity
- ❏ C   passing the wrong gas through it
- ❏ D   back pressure from the Manley ventilator
- ❏ E   using it at high altitude

2.78 The critical temperature is

- ❏ A   the temperature at which a gas becomes liquid if the pressure is raised
- ❏ B   the temperature above which a gas cannot be liquefied by increasing pressure alone
- ❏ C   the temperature at which latent heat of vaporisation equals zero
- ❏ D   the temperature that separates gases from vapours
- ❏ E   always lower than the boiling point of the same gas

2.79 A new anaesthetic agent has a saturated vapour pressure at 20°C of 152 mmHg. If there is a total fresh gas flow of 4 l/min, of which 80 ml is diverted through the vaporiser, the inspired concentration will be approximately

☐ A 1.6%
☐ B 0.8%
☐ C 2%
☐ D 0.4%
☐ E 5%

2.80 The critical pressure is

☐ A the maximum pressure to which a cylinder can be filled
☐ B the pressure above which a liquid cannot evaporate
☐ C the pressure at which vapour is in equilibrium with its liquid
☐ D 120 bar
☐ E the pressure at which a gas ignites

2.81 The following are true for gases in cylinders

☐ A oxygen is stored at 150 bar
☐ B nitrous oxide is stored at 137 bar
☐ C nitrous oxide should contain 1% water vapour
☐ D nitrous oxide should not be stored below −8°C
☐ E size E cylinders of oxygen and nitrous oxide are generally used on a Boyle's machine

2.82 For laminar flow in a tube, the flow rate is directionally proportional to

☐ A its length
☐ B the fourth power of its radius
☐ C the density of the gas or liquid flowing through it
☐ D the pressure drop across it
☐ E the viscosity of the gas or liquid flowing through it

2.83 The vapour pressure of a liquid

- ❏ A   is linearly related to temperature
- ❏ B   can exceed the normal atmospheric pressure
- ❏ C   is a function of barometric pressure
- ❏ D   maintains a constant percentage of the vapour in the gas phase in a closed space above the liquid irrespective of the total pressure
- ❏ E   determines the gram molecular volume of the vapour

2.84 Concerning fires and explosions in theatre

- ❏ A   the relative humidity in the theatre should be kept at about 55%
- ❏ B   air is safer than oxygen
- ❏ C   switches within the zone of risk should be spark proof
- ❏ D   the floor should be terrazzo on a well-conducting screed
- ❏ E   cotton fabrics are better than silk

2.85 Regarding the gas laws

- ❏ A   Boyle's law states that at a constant temperature, the volume of a given mass of gas varies directly with pressure
- ❏ B   Charles' law states that at a constant pressure, the volume of a given mass of gas varies directly with temperature
- ❏ C   they state that, at a constant volume, the absolute pressure of a given mass of gas varies indirectly with temperature
- ❏ D   they enable the pressure gauge to act as a contents gauge on the nitrous oxide cylinder
- ❏ E   in a mixture of gases, the pressure exerted by each of the gases is the same as it would exert if it alone occupied the cylinder

2.86 Regarding heat loss

- ❏ A   respiration accounts for 20% of heat loss
- ❏ B   radiation accounts for 40% of heat loss
- ❏ C   conduction accounts for 30% of heat loss
- ❏ D   more heat is lost humidifying than warming inspired gases
- ❏ E   the fall in temperature in the first hour of anaesthesia is 0.7°C if the theatre temperature is 21°C –24°C

2.87 Capnography

☐ A works on the absorption of carbon dioxide in the ultraviolet region of the spectrum

☐ B if used in combination with pulse oximetry, it would reduce anaesthetic mishaps by 90%

☐ C the P_aCO_2/P_eCO_2 gradient in a patient with V/Q mismatch is 0.7 kPa

☐ D collision broadening may occur in the presence of oxygen

☐ E there are two sampling methods: side and main stream

2.88 When using diathermy

☐ A a low-frequency current is used to maximise safety

☐ B the degree of burning depends on the current density

☐ C the likelihood of the patient sustaining a burn is reduced by using a large neutral plate

☐ D the spark gap determines whether the diathermy is used in the cutting or coagulation mode

☐ E if the neutral plate is disconnected, the patient may sustain a burn under the ECG electrodes

2.89 Regarding flow in a cylinder

☐ A if it is laminar, the flow will be directly proportional to the viscosity of the fluid

☐ B if it is turbulent, the flow will be indirectly proportional to the viscosity of the fluid

☐ C if the Reynolds' number is less than 2000, laminar flow is likely

☐ D if it is laminar, halving the diameter of the tube will reduce the flow by one-eighth

☐ E if it is turbulent, the flow will be directly proportional to the pressure across the tube

2.90 When using invasive blood pressure monitoring

❏   A   damping may be caused by clot formation in the cannula

❏   B   the resonant frequency may be increased by decreasing the compliance of the tubing

❏   C   the resonant frequency may be increased by increasing the width of the tubing

❏   D   if under-damped, the systolic and diastolic pressure will be overestimated

❏   E   the flow in the flushing system should exceed 4 ml/h so as to prevent clot formation

MCQ Paper 2 – Answers

2.1 Answers: A B D E

The dextrans are a group of branched polysaccharides produced by bacterial modification of sucrose. They improve peripheral blood flow by reducing blood viscosity and adhering to both the endothelium and cellular elements of blood, thus causing problems with the cross matching of blood. Impairing platelet activity as well as reducing levels of factor VIII reduce the risk of venous thrombosis. Side-effects include renal failure due to tubular obstruction in the kidney and anaphylactoid reactions, thought to be the result of previous cross-immunisation against bacterial antigens.

2.2 Answers: A D

Potassium is an intracellular ion released from myocytes during depolarisation following suxamethonium, raising the serum K transiently by 0.5 mmol/l in normal adults. Extensive tissue trauma will also release potassium from the cells, raising serum levels. Metabolic alkalosis will cause hypokalaemia following renal compensation. D-Tubocurarine, being a non-depolarising neuromuscular blocking agent, has no effect on serum K.

2.3 Answers: A E

Non-depolarising neuromuscular blocking agents are highly ionised compounds at body pH, exhibiting two quaternary ammonium groups. Their action is prolonged by hypothermia and severe acidosis. Monitoring of the blockade exhibits fade during 'train of four'; tetanic contraction also exhibits fade followed by post-tetanic facilitation. Depolarising neuromuscular blockade produces fasciculation and may exhibit dual block.

2.4 Answers: A D E

Although not generally available in the UK, ether is still used worldwide.

It is considered one of the safest of inhalational anaesthetics, largely because cardiovascular depression is late and is preceded by respiratory depression. However, postoperative convulsions often associated with pyrexia and prior atropine administration are recognised.

Once serum levels of bupivacaine exceed 2–4 mg/ml, either by misplacement of solution or excess dosage, central nervous system depression followed by convulsions may occur. Concurrently, there may be cardiovascular collapse. Suxamethonium produces muscle fasciculation and inhalational anaesthetics may all produce postoperative shivering, which is not to be confused with convulsions.

2.5   Answers: A B

Pain is not associated with intravenous injection of thiopentone, but should raise the possibility of intra-arterial injection or extravasation of the drug, both of which cause a severe burning sensation. Severe hypotension may occur especially following relative overdose or during hypovolaemia. Respiratory depression is common. Thiopentone induces liver enzymes but liver toxicity has not been reported.

2.6   Answers: A C D E

The boiling point of enflurane is 56.5°C compared with 50°C for halothane. Hypotension is more common with enflurane than halothane, due to greater myocardial depression and peripheral vasodilatation. Halothane causes greater sensitisation of the myocardium and therefore arrhythmias. Respiratory depression is greater with enflurane, reducing tidal volume and increasing respiratory rate. Both agents will release inorganic fluoride ions though the amount from halothane is negligible.

2.7   Answer: A

Digoxin is widely used to treat supraventricular arrhythmias such as atrial fibrillation (AF), atrial flutter and supraventricular tachycardia (SVT). Ventricular tachyarrhythmias are a feature of digoxin toxicity, which may be treated with phenytoin or digoxin-specific antibodies.

2.8   Answers: A C

Propranolol is a non-selective competitive antagonist at β1 and β2 receptors. It will therefore result in bronchoconstriction and reduced cardiac output in patients with bronchial hypersensitivity or cardiac impairment. By blocking β1 receptors it slows heart rate and may be used either alone or in conjunction with digoxin to slow the ventricular response in atrial fibrillation.

2.9 Answers: A B C

Dopamine is a naturally occurring catecholamine and neurotransmitter found in postganglionic sympathetic nerve endings and in the adrenal medulla. Its effects are dose-dependent. In doses up to 5 µg/kg per min, renal blood flow, GFR, urine output and sodium excretion (by impaired tubular reabsorption of Na^+ ions) are increased. At 10 µg/kg per min peripheral resistance is increased due to an action on α-adrenoreceptors. Although tachycardia is common, ventricular arrhythmias usually only occur at very high doses.

2.10 Answers: A D E

A derivative of phencyclidine, ketamine is metabolised in the liver to weakly active metabolites which are excreted in the urine.

Ketamine increases blood pressure and heart rate as well as cerebral blood flow and intracranial pressure (ICP). Muscular tone is enhanced as is uterine tone. Airway reflexes are maintained and, as salivation may be increased, pre-medication with an antisialagogue is recommended.

2.11 Answers: C D E

Sodium dantrolene is a skeletal muscle relaxant that directly affects excitation–contraction coupling within skeletal muscle by reducing the amount of calcium released by the sarcoplasmic reticulum. It has no effect on neuromuscular transmission, the membrane potential or muscle excitability itself. It is effective in treating malignant hyperpyrexia at a dose of 1–10 mg/kg.

2.12 Answers: A E

Isoflurane was first synthesised in 1965 along with its isomer enflurane, but not introduced until 1980 because of (subsequently unfounded) reports of carcinogenicity in rats. Its MAC is 1.15% and SVP at 20°C is 33 kPa, similar to halothane (32 kPa). Blood pressure is reduced mainly by peripheral vasodilatation, but at 1 MAC or less cerebral blood flow is not increased.

2.13 Answers: A C

Blood pressure and systemic vascular resistance are reduced by morphine mediated by histamine release. Miosis results from stimulation of the Edinger–Westphal nucleus and vomiting from stimulation of the chemoreceptor trigger zone in the floor of the IVth ventricle. Although there is a reduced ventilatory response to hypoxia and hypercapnia, at normal therapeutic dosages the arterial PCO_2 is not markedly raised.

2.14 Answers: A B C D E

The pharmacological effects of chlorpromazine are mediated by antagonism of histamine receptors, α-adrenergic receptors, central D2 dopaminergic receptors, muscarinic cholinergic receptors and serotoninergic receptors.

2.15 Answers: B D E

Chlorpropamide is a sulphonylurea, which stimulates insulin release from pancreatic β cells and increases the number and sensitivity of peripheral insulin receptors. It is extensively metabolised by the liver to a variety of active and inactive metabolites which are renally excreted. The elimination half-life of 27–39 hours may be markedly increased by renal impairment. Side-effects occur in around 6% of patients (compared with 3% of those taking tolbutamide) and include a disulfiram-like interaction when taken with alcohol.

2.16 Answers: A B E

The MAC of an inhalation anaesthetic agent, expressed in terms of % of one atmosphere, serves as a useful guide to clinical dosage as potency is inversely related to MAC. Potency is related to the oil/gas partition coefficient. MAC is reduced by other depressant drugs, including other anaesthetic agents, hypothermia, hypoxaemia and extremes of age. It is unaffected by sex, acid–base balance and hyper or hypocapnia.

2.17 Answers: A B C D E

Halothane produces a dose-dependent decrease in myocardial contractility and cardiac output mediated by inhibition of Ca ion flux within myocardial cells. The systemic vascular resistance is decreased by 15%–18% and the baroreceptor reflexes are obtunded.

It has ganglion-blocking and central vasomotor depressant actions all resulting in hypotension.

2.18 Answers: B E

Bupivacaine is a local anaesthetic which acts by diffusing through neural sheaths in the uncharged base form to combine with hydrogen ions, forming a cationic structure which is able to block the internal opening of the sodium ion channel, thereby preventing Na ion conductance and cell membrane depolarisation. The recommended maximal dose is 2 mg/kg. Metabolism occurs in the liver by N-dealkylation. Methaemoglobinaemia occurs with >600 mg administration of prilocaine.

2.19 Answers: A B C E

Chlorpropamide is an oral hypoglycaemic agent and has no anticonvulsant properties. Benzodiazepines and chlormethiazole act via facilitation of GABA receptors, opening chloride channels and hyperpolarising the cell membrane. Barbiturates also enhance chloride ion conductance but in the absence of GABA receptors.

2.20 Answers: A D E

Albumin is synthesised in the liver and forms a major constituent of plasma protein. It is important in maintenance of the plasma oncotic pressure. Normal values are 34–45 g/l. The plasma concentration is reduced in severe illness, infection, trauma, chronic liver disease and malabsorption.

2.21 Answers: B E

Neither atropine nor methylene blue causes methaemoglobinaemia.

Prilocaine in doses in excess of 600 mg may cause methaemoglobinaemia.

Levels of methaemoglobin should be monitored when using nitric oxide in acute respiratory distress syndrome (ARDS) patients. Cyanide ions will react with methaemoglobin to form cyanomethaemoglobin, ie they will reduce levels of methaemoglobin.

2.22 Answers: A C E

Cyclizine is thought to exert its anti-emetic action via blockade of H1 receptors centrally whilst hyoscine acts via antagonism of acetylcholine at muscarinic receptors. Perphenazine blocks D2 dopaminergic receptors whereas apomorphine, an alkaloid derived from morphine, has powerful dopamine agonist action causing intense stimulation of the chemoreceptor trigger zone and vomiting. Carbimazole inhibits thyroxine synthesis.

2.23 Answers: A B C D E

Although thiazide diuretics act mainly on the distal convoluted tubule, where they inhibit Na ion reabsorption, they also act at the proximal convoluted tubule causing weak inhibition of carbonic anhydrase and increasing bicarbonate and potassium excretion.

Side-effects include hypokalaemia, hyponatraemia, hyperuricaemia, hypomagnesaemia, hypochloraemia, hyperglycaemia, hyperchloraemic alkalosis and hypercholesterolaemia. Whilst loop diuretics promote calcium excretion and are used in the treatment of hypercalcaemia, thiazide diuretics cause calcium retention and increased serum calcium levels. Due to the effects on serum potassium and magnesium levels they may potentiate digoxin and increase the likelihood of digoxin toxicity.

2.24 Answers: C D E

Ketamine causes tachycardia, and an increase in blood pressure, central venous pressure and cardiac output secondary to an increase in sympathetic tone. Cerebral blood flow, intraocular and intracerebral pressure are all increased. Emergence delirium and hallucinations are common and reduced by benzodiazepine premedication.

Muscle hypertonia may require positioning of the patient prior to induction.

2.25 Answers: A C E

The effect of systemic or respiratory acidosis is to increase the potency and prolong the duration of action of non-depolarising neuromuscular blocking drugs. This may be either due to a direct effect of the pH on the physiochemical properties of these drugs or due to the concurrent effects on potassium metabolism, alkalosis promoting a shift of potassium into the cells raising the resting membrane potential and preventing depolarisation. Both hypermagnesaemia and hypocalcaemia will potentiate a competitive neuromuscular blockade due to their effects on the membrane potential.

2.26 Answers: A C D

Five cyanide ions are produced by the degradation of each nitroprusside molecule; one reacts with methaemoglobin to form cyanomethaemoglobin, the four remaining cyanide molecules enter the plasma, 80% of these react with thiosulphate in a reaction catalysed by hepatic rhodanese to form inactive thiocyanate. The remainder react with hydroxycobalamin to form cyanocobalamin. When these pathways are exhausted free cyanide ions are able to bind to cytochrome C, inhibiting aerobic metabolism and resulting in lactic acidosis. Toxicity is related to the rate of infusion rather than the total dose used, however it is recommended that no more than 1.5 mg/kg is infused acutely.

2.27 Answers: B C

Propranolol may mask the symptoms of hypoglycaemia but does not cause it per se. It is a competitive antagonist at β1 and β2 receptors resulting in bradycardia and bronchoconstriction.

Adrenergic receptor activity is mediated via cyclic AMP, as is enoximone, which is a phosphodiesterase inhibitor.

2.28 Answers: B C D

Frusemide acts by inhibition of active chloride ion reabsorption in the proximal tubule and ascending limb of the loop of Henle. By reducing the tonicity of the renal medulla, a hypotonic or isotonic urine is produced. This results in a diuresis and contraction of the circulating blood volume.

2.29 Answers: B D

Digoxin, verapamil and adenosine are used for supraventricular tachy-cardias, their site of action being the atrioventricular node.

Disopyramide acts at the level of the atria, ventricles and accessory pathways whereas lignocaine acts on the ventricles only. Both can be used to treat ventricular tachycardia.

2.30 Answers: A B

It is the partial pressure of an anaesthetic agent in the brain which is responsible for its anaesthetic effect. If an agent is insoluble in blood, little is removed from the alveoli by the pulmonary circulation and therefore the alveolar and brain partial pressure will rise rapidly. For agents with a high solubility, large amounts are removed from the alveoli, and increasing ventilation ensures a rapid replacement of the agent and increases the speed of induction. An increased cardiac output results in greater pulmonary blood flow, increasing uptake of the agent and therefore lowering alveolar partial pressure. Conversely, a low cardiac output will result in a reduced peripheral blood flow and blood returning to the lungs will still contain some anaesthetic agent. The partial pressure gradient between alveoli and blood is reduced, the net result being that alveolar concentration rises more rapidly.

2.31 Answers: A B C

In primary adrenal failure (Addison's disease) the anterior pituitary secretes adrenocorticotrophic hormone (ACTH) in response to stimulation by corticotrophin-releasing factor from the hypothalamus, but no cortisol or aldosterone is produced by the adrenal glands. ACTH, being similar to melatonin, produces hyperpigmentation of the skin creases. Lack of cortisol and aldosterone results in hypovolaemia, hyponatraemia, hypoglycaemia, hyperkalaemia and hypercalcaemia.

Treatment is with cortisol and aldosterone replacement therapy.

2.32 Answers: A B D E

Angiotensin II is produced from the action of angiotensin converting enzyme on angiotensin I in the lungs. It is a potent arteriolar vasoconstrictor which directly stimulates the thirst centre and releases aldosterone from the adrenal gland. The half-life of angiotensin II is 1–2 min and it is metabolised throughout the body including the lungs by a series of enzymes called angiotensinase.

2.33 Answers: B E

Gastrin is produced by the G cells in the lateral walls of the glands in the antral portion of the gastric mucosa. It is released in response to intra-luminal peptides or distension and vagal stimulation, which is mediated by gastrin releasing peptide and not acetylcholine.

Adrenaline due to sympathetic stimulation stimulates gastrin secretion and intraluminal acid provides the negative feedback loop to inhibit further gastrin production.

2.34 Answers: A C

Clearance is a calculated figure representing complete removal of a substance from plasma by passage through an organ, usually the kidney. In order to measure renal plasma flow the Fick principle may be applied. Since *para*-aminohippuric acid (PAH) is almost completely cleared by the kidney during one passage it is used to calculate renal plasma flow by determining steady-state plasma and urine concentrations.

Creatinine not urea is used to determine GFR, as following filtration it is neither reabsorbed nor secreted by the tubular cells. Inulin is filtered by the nephron but neither secreted nor reabsorbed, unlike glucose which is completely reabsorbed unless the renal threshold is exceeded. Water is reabsorbed in the distal collecting ducts under the control of ADH.

2.35 Answers: A C D

Physiological dead space equals anatomical plus alveolar dead space. The anatomical dead space comprises nose, mouth, pharynx and large airways not lined by respiratory epithelium. It is affected by posture, the size of the patient and increases with large respiratory efforts due to traction exerted on the bronchus by surrounding lung parenchyma. Alveolar dead space comprises the areas of the lung that are ventilated but not perfused.

2.36 Answer: D

Surfactant is produced by type II pneumocytes and forms a thin layer over the alveoli reducing the surface tension and increasing the compliance of the lung. One of the constituents of surfactant, dipalmitoyl phosphatidyl choline (DPPC), has hydrophobic and hydrophilic areas within the molecule which align themselves over the surface of the alveolus to exert their action.

2.37 Answers: B C D E

The pyramidal system consists of fibres running from area IV in the motor cortex to the contralateral motor nerves. The fibres form the pyramids in the medulla from where they gain their name and at which level 80%–90% decussate to form the lateral corticospinal tract of the spinal cord.

2.38 Answer: E

Both cardiac and smooth muscle cells, but not skeletal muscle, have low-resistance bridges between individual cells allowing them to act in a syncytial fashion. The resting membrane potential of skeletal and cardiac muscle is similar at –90 mV but smooth muscle has a much higher and more variable resting potential. The action potential duration is around 200 ms in cardiac muscle but shorter in smooth and skeletal muscle. Calcium influx from extracellular fluid is important in smooth muscle contraction, whereas in skeletal and cardiac myocytes calcium is released from the sarcoplasmic reticulum.

2.39 Answers: B C D E

The pulmonary vascular system is a distensible, low-pressure system. Pulmonary arterial pressure is around 25/9 mmHg with a mean pressure of 15 mmHg. In the normal erect subject 9% of the blood volume is in the pulmonary circulation, but this increases to 16% in the supine subject. Pulmonary vascular resistance is increased by adrenergic agonists, angiotensin II, thromboxanes and hypoxia. During exercise, pulmonary artery pressure is increased as is pulmonary blood flow; vascular resistance falls as previously closed portions of the vascular bed are recruited.

2.40 Answers: All false

Due to the patent ductus arteriosus and foramen ovale, the left and right sides of the heart pump in parallel in the fetus. At birth the systemic vascular resistance suddenly rises, the infant gasps, producing negative intrathoracic pressures of –40 to –50 cmH$_2$O.

Pulmonary vascular resistance falls and blood is pumped around the pulmonary circulation. Blood returning from the lungs raises the pressure in the left atrium, closing the foramen ovale and separating the two circulations. The ductus arteriosus constricts at birth and fuses completely within the first few days of life. Haemoglobin F persists until 3–4 months of age.

2.41 Answers: B C D E

Carbon dioxide is carried in the blood mainly as bicarbonate; 5%–10% dissolved in plasma and 5%–30% as carbamino compounds.

It is 20 times more soluble than oxygen and therefore crosses the placenta more easily. Deoxygenated haemoglobin can bind more carbon dioxide to form carbamino compounds thus facilitating loading of CO$_2$ in the peripheral capillaries.

2.42 Answers: C E

Emotional syncope is commonly due to abrupt vasodilatation combined with a reflex bradycardia. Sinus arrhythmia causes an increased heart rate on inspiration and slowing on expiration.

Noradrenaline infusion causes a bradycardia via increased blood pressure feeding back via the carotid sinus stretch receptors.

2.43 Answer: A

The carotid and to a lesser extent aortic bodies respond to reduced partial pressure (rather than content) of oxygen in arterial blood by stimulating ventilation. The central chemoreceptors respond to changes in pH and PCO_2, whilst the central respiratory neurones are depressed by hypoxia.

2.44 Answer: A

Muscle fibres are long multinucleate cells 50–70 μm in diameter and ranging in length from a few millimetres to a few centimetres.

Individual fibres have a single neural contact near the mid-point, from where the action potential travels along the sarcolemmal membrane and down the transverse tubules to initiate a contraction.

2.45 Answers: A C D

The dorsal root is also called the sensory root because it carries only sensory fibres. Neurones from peripheral sensory receptors enter the spinal cord via the dorsal horn. Two-thirds of these neurones synapse in the dorsal grey horn of the spinal cord, the other third pass up the cord to the gracile and cuneate nuclei. Sensory neurones form part of the pathway for reflex arcs and the monitoring of muscular tone via the muscle spindles. The preganglionic output to the autonomic nervous system travels in the ventral nerve root.

2.46 Answers: C D E

Haemoglobin is a protein made up of 4 subunits, each of which contains a haem moiety which may bind reversibly with oxygen.

Nearly all of the oxygen in blood is carried by red blood cells bound to haem. At 37°C the solubility of oxygen in plasma is 0.03 ml/l per mmHg partial pressure. This equates to approximately 0.3 ml of O_2 per 100 ml of plasma. Plasma is 1.8 times as viscous as water but the major determinant of blood viscosity is the haematocrit. Plasma skimming occurs when red cells tend to flow in the centre of vessels leaving relatively red-cell-poor blood at the periphery. Ninety-five percent of the glucose consumed by red blood cells is metabolised by anaerobic glycolysis.

2.47 Answers: A B C E

The carotid bodies are found bilaterally at the bifurcation of the internal and external carotid arteries. They are supplied with blood by a branch of the external carotid artery. The rich blood supply of 200 ml/100 g per min (compared with 84 ml/100 g per min for the myocardium) is so great that the arteriovenous O_2 difference is very small and capillary gas tensions are very close to those of the arterial system.

They respond to hypoxia, or to a rise in PCO_2 or H^+ concentration by stimulating respiration.

2.48 Answers: A C D

Forced expiration against a closed glottis after full inspiration, to generate a pressure of 40 mmHg for 10 seconds, was originally described as a technique for expelling pus from the middle ear. Normal subjects show 4 phases. I: an increase in intrathoracic pressure expels blood from thoracic vessels. II: decrease in BP due to reduction in venous return; activation of the baroreceptor reflex causes tachycardia and vasoconstriction, raising BP towards normal. III: further drop in BP as intrathoracic pressure suddenly drops, with pooling of blood in the pulmonary vessels. IV: overshoot, as compensatory mechanisms continue to operate with venous return restored. Increased BP causes bradycardia. The central venous pressure does increase in line with the increase in mouth pressure (a 7-mmHg rise for each 10-mmHg rise in mouth pressure). It is a useful bedside test of autonomic function.

2.49 Answers: C D E

CSF contains 50%–60% of blood glucose, has a lower pH than blood but will reflect changes in blood H^+ concentration. Seventy percent of CSF is formed by the choroid plexuses and absorbed via bulk flow into the arachnoid villi and cerebral blood vessels. Increased venous pressure will reduce the reabsorptive capacity.

2.50 Answers: B C

The ABO blood groups are inherited in a Mendelian fashion.

Donated blood is separated from plasma and resuspended in another medium prior to transfusion.

The characteristics of each blood group are as follows.

Phenotype	Genotype	Antigen on cells	Antibody in serum	Frequency (%)
A	AA, AO	A	Anti B	42
B	BB, BO	B	Anti A	8
AB	AB	A, B	None	3
O	OO	None	Anti A, Anti B	47

2.51 Answer: A

Acetylcholine is the transmitter at nicotinic receptors of the neuromuscular junction. Formed within the nerve terminal from choline and acetyl coenzyme A in the presence of choline transferase, it is released into the synaptic cleft where it is later hydrolysed by acetylcholinesterase. Botulinum toxin binds irreversibly to the nerve ending preventing acetylcholine release.

2.52 Answer: A

Enkephalin is an endogenous pentapeptide opioid agonist formed from proencephalon. It is found in the nerve endings of the gastrointestinal tract, adrenal, medulla and many different parts of the brain. It has a short half-life in the brain, terminated by metabolism by enkephalinase enzymes. Proopiomelanocortin, the precursor of endorphin, is primarily located in the hypothalamus and pituitary.

2.53 Answers: B C D

Tachycardia and an increase in the force of myocardial contraction are both due to β1 adrenergic agonism, mediated by increases in intracellular cAMP. Pupillary dilation is mediated via alpha agonism, which also produces vasoconstriction of splanchnic and visceral vessels. Vasodilatation in muscle and skin vessel beds is mediated via β2 and some β1 receptors.

2.54 Answers: B E

Glucocorticoids cause protein catabolism and increased hepatic glyco-genesis and gluconeogenesis. They have mild mineralocorticoid activity, promoting K+ loss and retaining salt and water.

They affect bone by promoting resorption and inhibiting formation, resulting in osteoporosis. Although cortisol feeds back on the anterior pituitary, inhibiting ACTH secretion, it does not depress other functions of the pituitary gland.

2.55 Answers: B D

Isotonic saline has the same osmolality as plasma and will cause plasma expansion without changing osmolality. Vasopressin reduces osmolality via water retention whilst aldosterone will increase osmolality via Na+ retention from sweat and salivary glands and in the kidney. Isotonic glucose will be rapidly metabolised resulting in a reduction in osmolality. Twenty percent albumin solution is hypertonic, drawing 3 times the administered volume into the circulation within 15 minutes.

2.56 Answers: A B C D E

Within a few minutes of TSH injection iodide binding is increased in the thyroid gland. Formation of T_3, T_4 and iodotyrosines are increased as well as secretion of thyroglobulin into the colloid. TSH effects its action via G proteins and cAMP.

2.57 Answer: E

Due to failure of exocrine and endocrine functions of the pancreas, both insulin and glucagon will decrease, impairing carbohydrate and fat metabolism and increasing plasma levels of free fatty acids.

Steatorrhoea is common due to the lack of pancreatic lipase.

2.58 Answers: A C

Glucagon is glycogenolytic, gluconeogenic, lipolytic and ketogenic. Glucose is formed from amino acids thus lowering plasma levels whilst free fatty acids are released. It exerts a positive inotropic and chronotropic action on the myocardium via increased myocardial calcium release, and has been used in the treatment of β adrenergic antagonist overdoses, though it does not stimulate the sympathetic nervous system directly.

2.59 Answers: A B

Both vasopressin and renin are secreted in response to a reduced extracellular fluid volume. Progesterone blocks the action of aldosterone. ACTH and thyroxine are unaffected.

2.60 Answer: E

High plasma calcium reduces intestinal absorption via reduction in 1,25-dihydroxycholecalciferol and formation of 24,25-dihydroxycholecalciferol instead. Calcitonin is increased, inhibiting bone reabsorption and increasing urinary Ca^{2+} excretion. Bone demineralisation may occur in the presence of primary hyperparathyroidism but is not directly due to hypercalcaemia itself.

2.61 Answers: A D

The Wright's respirometer is a vane anemometer. It measures volume by monitoring the continuous rotation of the vane as it is moved by the passing gas. It tends to over read at high tidal volumes and under read at low volumes as a result of the inertia of the vanes.

Moisture will cause the vanes to stick resulting in inaccurate readings.

2.62 Answers: A C D

The use of evoked potentials for monitoring the depth of anaesthesia or the integrity of the central nervous system during surgery involves monitoring the electrical activity produced by repetitive peripheral or central stimulation. Somatosensory, auditory and visually evoked potentials have all been used but they require complex equipment to increase the recording sensitivity and reduce background interference. Somatosensory-evoked potentials involve supramaximal stimulation usually of the tibialis or median nerves with simultaneous recording over the sensory area appropriate to the site of stimulation. Transmission is altered in the form of latency and amplitude of the signal with varying levels of anaesthesia.

2.63 Answers: A D

For accurate measurement of blood pressure it is essential that the width of the cuff should be in proportion to the size of the arm. The correct width is 20% greater than the width of the arm. Raising the arm above the level of the heart will result in a lower pressure being recorded. Slow cuff deflation and the position of the sphygmomanometer will not affect the reading.

2.64 Answer: B

Nitrogen at high pressure has a narcotic effect and this is the reason for the use of helium for diving to depths below 70 m. During normal respiration, with laminar gas flow, it is the viscosity of a gas that determines flow, however the viscosities of helium and nitrogen are similar. During turbulent flow the density of a gas becomes important; helium is less dense than nitrogen and it is for this reason that it is used as a carrier gas in cases of upper airway obstruction.

2.65 Answers: A B E

A current of as little as 150 μA delivered direct to the myocardium can induce ventricular fibrillation. The risk of electric current flowing along an intracardiac catheter is increased if it is filled with a conducting solution such as saline, likewise an oesophageal electrode can provide a low-resistance route for the delivery of current to the myocardium. Multiple earth loops will increase the likelihood of current flowing through the patient from any faulty equipment. Connection of equipment casing to earth, double insulation of conducting wire within equipment and the use of isolated circuits are all measures taken to try to avoid microshock.

2.66 Answers: A C

The Fick principle relates blood flow to an organ in unit time to the amount of marker substance taken up by that organ in that time and the concentration difference of the substance in vessels supplying and draining the organ. For cardiac output the oxygen consumption by the lungs together with arterial and mixed venous oxygen contents are used.

Cardiac output (l/min) = O_2 consumption (ml/min)/arterial-mixed venous O_2 concentration (ml/l).

2.67 Answers: A B E

Nitrous oxide is produced by heating ammonium nitrate above 240°C. Ammonia, nitric acid, nitrogen, nitric oxide and nitrogen dioxide are also produced. Ammonia and nitric acid reconstitute to form ammonium nitrate; nitric oxide and nitrogen dioxide pass through a series of scrubbers to ensure they are completely removed, as both are highly toxic. Carbon dioxide is formed by heating calcium or magnesium carbonate. Helium is obtained from natural gas. Oxygen concentrators compress and cool air then remove water vapour by passing through silicone gel, and nitrogen by passing through zeolite-filled cylinders. They can provide 90%–95% oxygen at up to 4 l/min, however 2–5% argon is present in the final mixture.

2.68 Answers: C D

In an exponential process the rate of change of a quantity at any time is proportional to the quantity at that time. The half-life is the time taken for the initial quantity to fall to half its original value. The time constant is the time in which the process would have been completed had the initial rate of change continued unchanged.

Consequently the time constant is longer than the half-life. After one time constant 63% of the change is completed, leaving 37% remaining.

2.69 Answers: A B C E

Airway resistance is the pressure difference between the alveoli and the mouth divided by the flow rate. Mouth pressure can be measured using a water-filled manometer and alveolar pressure can be deduced from measurements made in a body plethysmograph.

Airway resistance is increased at low lung volumes due to the reduction of radial traction produced by the lung parenchyma. Thus airway resistance is increased by anaesthesia due to reduced lung volume, though inhalational anaesthetics per se reduce resistance via a bronchodilator action. Positive end-expiratory pressure will increase lung volume and reduce airway resistance.

2.70 Answers: A E

The single-breath nitrogen test is used to measure anatomical dead space by following the nitrogen concentration at the mouth after a single inspiration of 100% oxygen. N_2 concentration rises as dead space gas is increasingly washed out by alveolar gas. Pure alveolar gas forms a plateau concentration of nitrogen, then towards the end of expiration an abrupt increase in N_2 concentration is seen. This is the closing volume caused by preferential emptying of the apex of the lung, which has a relatively higher N_2 concentration.

Distribution of gas delivery in the lung is measured with xenon and diffusion capacity with carbon monoxide.

2.71 Answers: A C D E

The alveolar arterial gradient is an indicator of the exchange properties of the lung. It depends on diffusion across the alveolar membrane and physiological shunt. If the closing capacity exceeds the functional residual capacity there will be increased ventilation/perfusion (V/Q) mismatch and shunting. In the elderly the closing capacity rises, often exceeding the functional residual capacity during normal tidal volume breathing, resulting in V/Q mismatch.

2.72 Answers: B C D

Commercial oxygen is produced by fractional distillation of air. Its boiling point is $-183°C$ and the critical temperature is $-118°C$.

Exposure to hyperbaric oxygen produces increased oxygen dissolved in blood but no increase in the amount of oxygen carried by haemoglobin, which is usually almost fully saturated. Symptoms evoked by hyperbaric oxygen are tracheobronchial irritation, dizziness, nausea, ringing in the ears, convulsions and coma. Bone marrow depression occurs following prolonged exposure to nitrous oxide.

2.73 Answers: B C E

Nitrous oxide is a vapour at room temperature as this is below its critical temperature of $36.5°C$. Nitrous oxide cylinders are filled with a combination of liquid and gaseous nitrous oxide. If completely filled with liquid any increase in temperature would cause a dangerous rise in pressure within the cylinder; therefore nitrous oxide cylinders are only partially filled with liquid according to the filling ratio. The pressure gauge relates to the amount of nitrous oxide in the gaseous phase, and is not therefore a reliable indicator of the amount remaining in the cylinder until all the liquid has been exhausted. Higher oxides of nitrogen are produced during the heating of ammonium nitrate to form nitrous oxide. They can be tested for with moistened starch-iodide paper, which will turn blue in the presence of nitric oxide or nitrogen dioxide.

2.74 Answers: C D E

The approximate composition of soda lime is 90% calcium hydroxide, 5% sodium hydroxide and 1% potassium hydroxide with silicates for binding and an indicator. The moisture content is 14%–19%, which is essential for effective carbon dioxide absorption.

Carbon dioxide in solution reacts with sodium and potassium hydroxide to form the respective carbonates, which then react with calcium hydroxide to produce calcium carbonate, replenishing sodium and potassium hydroxide. In a properly packed canister half the volume should be space between the granules. Heat is produced by the chemical reaction that takes place.

2.75 Answers: A B C

The Magill circuit is an example of a Mapleson type A, the coaxial modification of which is called the Lack circuit. The effort required to open the expiratory valve precludes its use in small children but it is suitable for those weighing more than 20 kg. During spontaneous ventilation exhaled dead space is retained, to be inhaled at the next inspiration, whereas exhaled alveolar gas is vented through the expiratory valve. Therefore fresh gas flow may be reduced to alveolar ventilation (normally about 70% of minute ventilation) before rebreathing will occur.

2.76 Answers: A B C D

The central venous pressure is usually measured with the patient lying flat, and expressed in cmH_2O above a fixed point level with the right atrium, eg the mid axillary line. Alterations in the position of the patient will affect the measurement as will wetting the manometer tube plug. During normal spontaneous breathing the pressure falls on inspiration and rises on expiration. Large negative intrathoracic pressures such as those generated by patients with airway obstruction will accentuate the fall and cause inaccuracies in central venous pressure measurement.

2.77 Answers: A B C D E

Dirt on the bobbin or static electricity may cause the bobbin to stick to the glass tubing of the rotameter. Ventilators which exert back pressure such as the Manley will depress the level of the bobbin and errors of up to 7% may result. Rotameters are calibrated for an individual bobbin and a specific gas at sea level, changes in the type of gas or barometric pressure will lead to inaccuracy.

2.78 Answers: A B D

The critical temperature is defined as the temperature above which a substance cannot be liquefied however much pressure is applied.

The critical pressure is the vapour pressure of a substance at its critical temperature. The word 'gas' applies to a substance above its critical temperature while 'vapour' is the word used for a substance below its critical temperature. At room temperature oxygen and nitrogen are gases whilst nitrous oxide, carbon dioxide and halothane are vapours.

2.79 Answer: D

As the saturated vapour pressure is 152 mmHg then at atmospheric pressure (760 mmHg) the gas passing through the chamber will be approximately 20% saturated (152/760). As 2% of total gas flow passes through the chamber (80 ml/4 l) then the inspired concentration is 0.4%.

2.80 Answers: All false

The critical pressure is the vapour pressure of a substance at its critical temperature.

2.81 Answer: E

The pressure within oxygen and Entonox cylinders is 137 bar, nitrous oxide is stored at 40 bar. Entonox should not be stored at −8°C as this is below the pseudocritical temperature at which separation of the gases will occur, allowing the possibility of delivering a hypoxic mixture of oxygen/nitrous oxide.

2.82 Answers: B D

According to the Hagen–Poiseuille equation regarding laminar flow:

Gas flow = $[\pi(P_1-P_2)\cdot r^4]/8\mu l$.

where (P_1-P_2) is the pressure drop, μ the viscosity and l the length of the tube. Density becomes important only in turbulent flow.

2.83 Answers: A E

The vapour pressure is the pressure exerted by molecules escaping from the surface of a liquid to enter the gaseous phase. When equilibrium is reached at any temperature, the number of molecules leaving the liquid equals the number re-entering it; the vapour pressure now equals the saturated vapour pressure (SVP). Raising the temperature increases the kinetic energy of the molecules allowing more to escape to the gaseous phase and raising the SVP. When SVP equals barometric pressure the liquid boils.

2.84 Answers: A B C D E

Fires and explosions occur when a substance combines with oxygen or other oxidising agent with the release of energy.

Activation energy is required to start the process, which may be provided from sparks from electrical equipment or static electricity from clothing, shoes or work surfaces. The risk of accumulation of static electricity on walls and equipment is reduced if the relative humidity is kept high. Floors of operating theatres are made of conductive materials to allow any build up of static charge to be safely drained away.

2.85 Answers: B E

For an ideal gas, $PV = nRT$ where P is the pressure, V is volume, n is the number of moles of gas, R is the universal gas constant and T is temperature. Nitrous oxide is a vapour at room temperature. The contents of a cylinder of nitrous oxide at 40 bar are therefore a mixture of liquid and gas.

2.86 Answers: B D E

General anaesthesia inhibits the patient's ability to maintain body temperature by depressing the thermoregulatory centre in the hypothalamus. Conductive losses are of little importance in air, but become highly significant when water is the conducting medium.

Respiratory losses account for 10% of heat loss of which 8% is due to the latent heat of vaporisation of water and 2% due to the heating of air. The temperature of a patient will rapidly fall following induction of general anaesthesia if no active warming measures are taken.

2.87 Answers: B E

Capnography is the continuous measurement and display of carbon dioxide in exhaled gas. It approximates to the alveolar partial pressure of carbon dioxide in normal subjects, however the normal P_aCO_2/P_eCO_2 gradient is 0.7 kPa and this will be increased by significant V/Q mismatch. Carbon dioxide absorbs infrared radiation within the sampling chamber of the capnograph. In the presence of nitrous oxide, carbon dioxide molecules may transfer some of this absorbed energy, causing broadening of the absorption spectrum of nitrous oxide. Side stream capnographs withdraw a sample of exhaled gas from a connector at the patient's airway, resulting in a timing delay. Mainstream analysers are connected at the patient's airway and therefore have no transit time delay.

2.88 Answers: B C E

Diathermy is used to coagulate blood vessels and cut and destroy tissues during surgical procedures. It is the heating effect of a high density of current which causes this effect at the site of action.

Normally high-frequency (0.5–1.0 MHz) alternating current is used as lower frequencies are more likely to induce ventricular fibrillation. A sine wave pattern is used for cutting and a pulsed sine wave for coagulation. The current density is kept high at the site of intended damage, the forceps tips, but low at the large surface area plate which acts as the other electrode. Incorrect attachment of the plate may cause increased current density and burns in the area, or the current may escape via an alternative route such as via ECG electrodes.

2.89 Answer: C

$Q=[\pi(P_1-P_2)\cdot r^4]/8\mu l$.

According to the Hagen–Poiseuille equation, during conditions of laminar flow halving the diameter of the tube reduces the flow by one-sixteenth (ie the fourth power) of its original value. Viscosity is inversely proportional to flow under these conditions. When the Reynolds' number exceeds 2000 turbulent flow is likely. Under these conditions flow is no longer proportional to the pressure drop and the density of a fluid becomes an important factor in determining flow.

2.90 Answers: A B C D E

Damping of biological systems involves the progressive diminution of amplitude of oscillations in a resonant system. Excess damping, due to air bubbles, clots or kinking within the system, results in a flattened trace. Optimal damping is defined as 0.6–0.7 of critical damping, producing a fast response without excessive oscillations.

Using a shorter, stiffer, wider catheter may increase the resonant frequency of the system. Continuous flushing at rates of 3–4 ml/h is preferable to intermittent flushing which may promote intimal damage and subsequent arterial thrombosis.

Multiple Choice Question Paper 3

90 Questions: time allowed 3 hours.

Indicate your answers with a tick or cross in the spaces provided.

3.1 The following antibiotics act by inhibiting cell wall synthesis

- ❑ A cephalosporins
- ❑ B tetracyclines
- ❑ C aminoglycosides
- ❑ D penicillins
- ❑ E sulphonamides

3.2 L-Dopa

- ❑ A is a metabolic product of dopamine
- ❑ B penetrates the CNS poorly
- ❑ C is not metabolised in peripheral tissues
- ❑ D can cause nausea
- ❑ E can cause arrhythmias

3.3 Propofol

- ❑ A is formulated in propylene glycol
- ❑ B has a pH greater than 10
- ❑ C is conjugated to glucuronides and sulphates in the liver
- ❑ D causes coronary vasodilatation
- ❑ E has a low hepatic clearance

3.4 The effects of α2-adrenoreceptor agonists include

- ❑ A sedation
- ❑ B a dry mouth
- ❑ C cold extremities
- ❑ D bradycardia
- ❑ E reduced analgesic requirements

3.5   Drugs may produce hypotension by an action on

- ❏   A   parasympathetic ganglia
- ❏   B   α adrenoreceptors
- ❏   C   β adrenoreceptors
- ❏   D   noradrenaline synthesis
- ❏   E   noradrenaline release

3.6   Tricyclic antidepressants

- ❏   A   inhibit neuronal uptake of noradrenaline
- ❏   B   have a rapid onset of action
- ❏   C   may cause a dry mouth and constipation
- ❏   D   do not produce postural hypotension
- ❏   E   may produce tachycardia and palpitations

3.7   Ketamine

- ❏   A   is a racemic mixture
- ❏   B   increases cardiac output
- ❏   C   has an action at NMDA-controlled ion channels
- ❏   D   induces anaesthesia in one arm brain circulation time
- ❏   E   has active metabolites

3.8   The following are potassium sparing

- ❏   A   frusemide
- ❏   B   amiloride
- ❏   C   triamterene
- ❏   D   acetazolamide
- ❏   E   spironolactone

3.9   β adrenoreceptor blocking drugs

- ❏   A   increase myocardial oxygen consumption
- ❏   B   may have partial agonist activity
- ❏   C   may have a quinidine-like effect
- ❏   D   may reduce hepatic blood flow
- ❏   E   reduce maximal exercise capacity

3.10 The blood–brain barrier is readily crossed by

- ❏ A glycopyrrolate
- ❏ B hyoscine
- ❏ C neostigmine
- ❏ D D-tubocurarine
- ❏ E morphine

3.11 Diazepam

- ❏ A has a longer terminal half-life in the elderly
- ❏ B is metabolised to midazolam
- ❏ C acts in the same time as thiopentone
- ❏ D increases GABA concentrations in the brain
- ❏ E is well absorbed following intramuscular injection

3.12 With regard to pharmacokinetics

- ❏ A zero-order kinetics indicates metabolism at a constant rate
- ❏ B first-order kinetics can change to zero-order kinetics
- ❏ C a three-compartment model is a feature of fat-soluble drugs
- ❏ D drugs with large volumes of distribution have long half-lives
- ❏ E compartments refer to anatomical structures

3.13 In severe liver disease

- ❏ A tubocurarine is potentiated
- ❏ B suxamethonium is potentiated
- ❏ C gallamine is potentiated
- ❏ D neostigmine is ineffective
- ❏ E atracurium is unaffected

3.14 The following drugs are more than 50% protein bound

- ❏ A phenytoin
- ❏ B morphine
- ❏ C diazepam
- ❏ D atracurium
- ❏ E alfentanil

3.15 The following dilate the pupil

- ❏ A   neostigmine
- ❏ B   cocaine
- ❏ C   ganglion blockers
- ❏ D   atenolol
- ❏ E   codeine

3.16 The following are metabolised by cholinesterase

- ❏ A   procaine
- ❏ B   neostigmine
- ❏ C   mivacurium
- ❏ D   suxamethonium
- ❏ E   diamorphine

3.17 The following show zero-order kinetics at normal doses

- ❏ A   phenytoin
- ❏ B   morphine
- ❏ C   aspirin
- ❏ D   ethyl alcohol
- ❏ E   warfarin

3.18 Sodium nitroprusside

- ❏ A   acts via nitric oxide
- ❏ B   causes tachycardia
- ❏ C   should be protected from light
- ❏ D   lowers intracranial pressure
- ❏ E   increases pulmonary artery pressure

3.19 The clearance of a drug

- ❏ A   represents the removal of a given amount of drug in unit time
- ❏ B   represents the rate of elimination per unit concentration in blood
- ❏ C   equals the volume of distribution multiplied by the half-life
- ❏ D   equals the volume of distribution multiplied by a constant
- ❏ E   is inversely proportional to the half-life

3.20 The following have an elimination half-life of more than 24 hours

❏ A   diazepam
❏ B   amiodarone
❏ C   chlorpropamide
❏ D   digoxin
❏ E   thiopentone

3.21 Coronary blood flow

❏ A   in health is affected by small (< 20 mmHg) changes in mean arterial BP
❏ B   is equal to diastolic blood pressure
❏ C   is mainly under humoral control
❏ D   increases following beta blockade by a direct vasodilator effect
❏ E   return is above 85% to the right atrium via the coronary sinus

3.22 In starvation

❏ A   muscle glycogen and brain glycogen are replenished by gluconeogenesis
❏ B   ketone bodies produced in the liver from free fatty acids can be utilised by brain cells, but glucose is still essential
❏ C   FFA oxidation in liver, muscle and heart is increased
❏ D   there is a fall in body potassium
❏ E   secondary to vomiting in children, the odour of breath is due to ketosis

3.23 The rate at which the alveolar concentration of an anaesthetic agent approaches the inspired concentration is a function of

❏ A   alveolar ventilation
❏ B   water solubility
❏ C   cardiac output
❏ D   saturated vapour pressure
❏ E   inspired concentration

3.24 In metabolic acidosis

- ❏ A base excess is positive
- ❏ B plasma bicarbonate never exceeds 30 mmol/l
- ❏ C standard bicarbonate falls
- ❏ D P_aCO_2 may be normal
- ❏ E urine pH falls

3.25 The following are features of an active transport system

- ❏ A expenditure of energy
- ❏ B independence from temperature
- ❏ C unaffected by hypoxia
- ❏ D movement against a concentration gradient
- ❏ E maximal transport rate

3.26 Iron

- ❏ A absorption is dependent on erythropoietin
- ❏ B absorption is dependent on total body iron
- ❏ C is carried in the plasma as transferrin
- ❏ D absorption requires an intact colonic mucosa
- ❏ E accumulation can result in a raised blood glucose

3.27 In a subject lying on his side breathing quietly

- ❏ A blood flow is greater in the lower lung
- ❏ B ventilation is greater in the lower lung
- ❏ C blood leaving the lower lung comes from an area with a higher V/Q than that leaving the upper lung
- ❏ D P_aO_2 is greater in blood coming from the lower lung
- ❏ E P_aCO_2 is greater in blood coming from the lower lung

3.28 On changing from standing to supine

- ❏ A heart rate increases
- ❏ B pressure in the leg veins increases
- ❏ C capacitance of the pulmonary veins increases
- ❏ D baroreceptor activity increases
- ❏ E there is a diuresis

3.29 The following are neurotransmitters at autonomic ganglia

- ❑ A histamine
- ❑ B bradykinin
- ❑ C adrenaline
- ❑ D methacholine
- ❑ E dopamine

3.30 During quiet inspiration

- ❑ A alveolar volume increases by 30%
- ❑ B abdominal muscles are active
- ❑ C sacrospinalis muscles are active
- ❑ D intrathoracic pressure decreases by a few mmHg
- ❑ E the ribcage does not move

3.31 Immediately after transection of the spinal cord in the cervical region the following are seen

- ❑ A loss of bladder reflexes
- ❑ B hypotension
- ❑ C loss of the knee reflex
- ❑ D spastic paralysis
- ❑ E loss of sensation in the legs

3.32 The sensation of pain

- ❑ A is conveyed mainly in the dorsal column
- ❑ B is augmented by β-endorphin
- ❑ C can be modified by cutting the spinothalamic tract
- ❑ D can be modified by strenuous exercise
- ❑ E can be modified by non-painful stimuli of the same area

3.33 Increased gamma motor neurone activity will result in

- ❑ A skeletal muscle relaxation
- ❑ B uterine contraction
- ❑ C vasodilatation
- ❑ D increased tone of voluntary muscles
- ❑ E hyperactive tendon reflexes

3.34 Concerning fetal circulation

☐ A   it is possible for vena caval blood to reach the aorta without going through the left ventricle or left atrium

☐ B   the P_aO_2 in the descending aorta is less than in the ductus arteriosus

☐ C   foramen ovale closes at birth because of the increased left atrial pressure

☐ D   flow in the ductus arteriosus stops/reverses at birth because of decreased pulmonary vascular resistance

☐ E   highly oxygenated blood reaches the head of the fetus via the right ventricle

3.35 The following influence aldosterone

☐ A   surgical stress
☐ B   high sodium intake
☐ C   renal ischaemia
☐ D   angiotensin
☐ E   plasma potassium concentration

3.36 The physiological response to haemorrhagic shock consists of

☐ A   increased sympathetic activity
☐ B   production of renin
☐ C   increased production of erythropoietin
☐ D   increased baroreceptor activity
☐ E   increased chemoreceptor activity

3.37 In the Valsalva manoeuvre there is

☐ A   an initial rise in blood pressure
☐ B   an initial tachycardia followed by bradycardia
☐ C   a fall in cardiac output
☐ D   an increase in renal blood flow
☐ E   an abnormal response in diabetics

3.38 Potassium

- [ ] A   excretion is increased by aldosterone
- [ ] B   normal excretion is up to 100 mmol/day
- [ ] C   excretion is decreased for up to 2–3 days postoperatively
- [ ] D   is filtered by the glomerulus
- [ ] E   is actively absorbed in the proximal tubule and loop of Henle

3.39 The intrinsic clotting cascade is associated with

- [ ] A   factor IX
- [ ] B   factor VII
- [ ] C   a faster speed of action than the extrinsic system
- [ ] D   initial activation of factor VIII
- [ ] E   an enzyme cascade

3.40 Cerebrospinal fluid (CSF)

- [ ] A   volume is 20% of intracranial volume
- [ ] B   pressure pulsates with blood pressure and respiration
- [ ] C   production is 0.4 mg/min from the choroid plexus
- [ ] D   is absorbed from the arachnoid villi
- [ ] E   pressure follows cerebral blood flow in the short term

3.41 The following can be used for the measurement of temperature

- [ ] A   the Seebeck effect
- [ ] B   alcohol thermometers
- [ ] C   mercury thermometers
- [ ] D   resistance
- [ ] E   interferometer

3.42 Concerning the sterilisation of anaesthetic equipment

- [ ] A   boiling in water for 15 min at atmospheric pressure kills bacteria and spores
- [ ] B   an autoclave pressure of 1 bar at a temperature of 120°C for 15 min will kill all living organisms
- [ ] C   ethylene oxide is only bactericidal
- [ ] D   ethylene oxide takes 2–4 hours to be completely effective
- [ ] E   a 0.1% solution of chlorhexidine will sterilise an endotracheal tube in 3 min

3.43 Minimum alveolar concentration (MAC)

- ❏ A is an index of potency of intravenous anaesthetics
- ❏ B is measured in volume %
- ❏ C can be determined by probit analysis
- ❏ D is affected by age
- ❏ E is a correlate of oil/water solubility

3.44 Measurement of airway resistance may entail the use of

- ❏ A an oesophageal balloon
- ❏ B body plethysmography
- ❏ C a pneumotachograph
- ❏ D a stethograph
- ❏ E a Haldane alveolar tube

3.45 Basal metabolic rate

- ❏ A is 70 kJ/m^2 per h
- ❏ B may be measured using an ergometer
- ❏ C is high in tropical climates
- ❏ D is low in children
- ❏ E is always elevated in patients with a goitre

3.46 Plasma volume can be measured using

- ❏ A *para*-aminohippuric acid
- ❏ B inulin
- ❏ C radioactively labelled albumin
- ❏ D Evans' blue
- ❏ E creatinine

3.47 Oxygen rotameters

- ❏ A can be used with nitrous oxide
- ❏ B consist of a bulb in a cylinder
- ❏ C are affected by back pressure
- ❏ D have a linear scale
- ❏ E are an example of a variable-orifice flowmeter

3.48 Pressure can be expressed as

- ❏ A force per unit area
- ❏ B kg/m/s² (kg·m⁻¹·s⁻²)
- ❏ C pascals
- ❏ D newton/m² (N·m⁻²)
- ❏ E bars

3.49 A paramagnetic gas analyser is useful for the measurement of

- ❏ A halothane
- ❏ B oxygen
- ❏ C nitrogen
- ❏ D nitrous oxide
- ❏ E carbon dioxide

3.50 Resistance to current flow in a wire changes with

- ❏ A tension in the wire
- ❏ B temperature in the wire
- ❏ C length of the wire
- ❏ D diameter of the wire
- ❏ E changes in the potential difference

3.51 Viscosity

- ❏ A decreases as the temperature of a gas increases
- ❏ B of a liquid rises as its temperature rises
- ❏ C is dependent on molecular cohesiveness
- ❏ D is dependent on Van der Waal's forces
- ❏ E of oxygen/helium mixtures is less than that of oxygen/nitrous oxide mixtures

3.52 Surface tension

- ❏ A changes with temperature
- ❏ B can be measured in pascal metres
- ❏ C is due to molecular cohesion
- ❏ D leads to a mercury manometer over-reading
- ❏ E depends on viscosity

3.53 According to Boyle's law

- ❏ A $PV = k$
- ❏ B 1 gram mol occupies 22.4 litres at room temperature
- ❏ C a plot of P versus V is a straight line
- ❏ D a plot of P versus V is a rectangular hyperbola
- ❏ E a plot of V versus P gives a reciprocal of k

3.54 The following disadvantages apply to these methods of temperature measurement

- ❏ A mercury in a glass thermometer has a slow response time
- ❏ B platinum resistance thermometer probes are not interchangeable
- ❏ C platinum resistance thermometer probes have a slow response time
- ❏ D thermistors can become unstable over a period of a few months
- ❏ E thermocouples have so many disadvantages that they are not in clinical use

3.55 Gas or air can be satisfactorily humidified in the following ways

- ❏ A passage through the upper respiratory tract
- ❏ B passage through a cold water bath
- ❏ C using the Bernoulli effect
- ❏ D using heated-water humidifiers
- ❏ E using the Joule Thompson effect

3.56 The following are properties of nitrous oxide

- ❏ A a boiling point of –8°C
- ❏ B nitrous oxide cylinders have a filling ratio of 0.9
- ❏ C helium and nitrous oxide can be used in the same flowmeter
- ❏ D a MAC value greater than 100%
- ❏ E a critical temperature of 36.5°C

3.57 In the measurement of CVP

- ❏ A the catheter must be less than 20 cm long
- ❏ B the ideal catheter diameter is greater than 0.25 cm
- ❏ C the reference point must be the angle of Louis
- ❏ D the patient must be lying flat
- ❏ E the ventilator should be disconnected when taking the CVP reading

3.58 The amount of gas that will dissolve in a liquid is determined by

❏ A temperature
❏ B ambient pressure
❏ C liquid
❏ D gas/liquid coefficient
❏ E molecular weight of the gas but not of the liquid

3.59 Spirometry can be used to measure

❏ A functional residual capacity (FRC)
❏ B total lung capacity (TLC)
❏ C residual volume (RV)
❏ D expiratory reserve volume
❏ E functional inspiratory reserve volume

3.60 Concerning the location of vaporisers within the anaesthetic circuit

❏ A with the vaporiser inside a circle (VIC), the inflow gas contains an unknown concentration of volatile agent
❏ B with VIC, an accurate vaporiser, efficient at low flows, should be used to maintain an accurate vapour flow within the circuit
❏ C with the vaporiser outside the circle (VOC) an inefficient vaporiser is adequate because inspired concentrations are not critical
❏ D with VOC, the anaesthetic vapour concentration within the circuit is dependent upon uptake
❏ E with VIC and low fresh gas flow, the inspired concentration is greater than the vaporiser setting

3.61 The following are equivalent to a pressure of one atmosphere

❏ A 100 mmHg
❏ B 1000 cmH$_2$O
❏ C 760 bar
❏ D 12 torr
❏ E 10 kPa

3.62 An intra-aortic balloon pump will increase

- ❑ A   heart rate
- ❑ B   myocardial workload
- ❑ C   coronary perfusion pressure
- ❑ D   left ventricular work
- ❑ E   left ventricular afterload

3.63 Concerning pacemakers and anaesthesia

- ❑ A   a magnet placed over a demand pacemaker will convert it to a fixed rate pacemaker
- ❑ B   unipolar diathermy should be used
- ❑ C   a patient with a pacemaker may safely enter an MRI scanner
- ❑ D   postoperative shivering may affect pacemaker function
- ❑ E   induction of anaesthesia may alter pacemaker function

3.64 Entonox

- ❑ A   is stored in cylinders at 137 bar
- ❑ B   has a pseudocritical temperature of ~ −7°C
- ❑ C   can be administered by registered midwives
- ❑ D   can lead to megaloblastic anaemia after prolonged exposure
- ❑ E   is a 50:50 mixture of nitric oxide and oxygen

3.65 With regard to Tuohy needles and epidural catheters

- ❑ A   the filter has pores of 22 μm diameter
- ❑ B   the standard needle is 16 gauge
- ❑ C   the needle is 10 cm long
- ❑ D   hanging drop technique may be used to locate the epidural space
- ❑ E   Lee markings are present at 1-cm intervals on the Tuohy needle

3.66 In an exponential process

- ❑ A   37% of the process is completed in one time constant
- ❑ B   95% of the process is completed in three time constants
- ❑ C   the rate of change is constant
- ❑ D   washout curves are exponential processes
- ❑ E   time constant and half-life are synonymous

3.67 Helium

- ❏ A   is stored as a liquid
- ❏ B   is a useful treatment for bronchospasm
- ❏ C   has similar viscosity to oxygen
- ❏ D   supports combustion
- ❏ E   is a narcotic at pressure

3.68 Wright's respirometer

- ❏ A   is inaccurate at flows of <1 l/min
- ❏ B   is a turbine
- ❏ C   is affected by viscosity of gas
- ❏ D   is affected by humidity
- ❏ E   can be used to measure peak flow

3.69 Peak flow

- ❏ A   is not effort dependent
- ❏ B   is measured by the pneumotachograph
- ❏ C   is measured by the vitalograph
- ❏ D   is reduced in acute asthma
- ❏ E   has a diurnal variation

3.70 The Severinghaus electrode

- ❏ A   consists of CO_2-sensitive glass
- ❏ B   is better with gases than with blood
- ❏ C   measures pH
- ❏ D   is affected by nitrous oxide
- ❏ E   contains bicarbonate ions in the electrolyte solution

3.71 Soda lime

- ❏ A   contains 70% calcium hydroxide and 30% sodium hydroxide
- ❏ B   may not be used with desflurane
- ❏ C   may warm to 60°C during active CO_2 absorption
- ❏ D   use has been associated with methaemoglobinaemia
- ❏ E   produces humidification of inspired gases

3.72 An arterial line in the radial artery can lead to

- ❏ A fatal haemorrhage
- ❏ B pulmonary embolism
- ❏ C intracerebral embolism
- ❏ D paraesthesia at the base of the thumb
- ❏ E septicaemia

3.73 The thromboelastograph (TEG)

- ❏ A will be a flat line if a heparinised sample is used
- ❏ B provides information about platelet function
- ❏ C provides information about thrombolysis
- ❏ D can be used to determine what blood products a bleeding patient may require
- ❏ E is much slower than laboratory estimation of PT, aPTT and platelet count

3.74 Transoesophageal echo (TOE)

- ❏ A can be used to assess cardiac output
- ❏ B employs ultrasound
- ❏ C is a very sensitive detector of pulmonary emboli
- ❏ D cannot be used with diathermy
- ❏ E is a Doppler probe

3.75 The hazard of microshock can be reduced by the use of

- ❏ A saline-filled intracardiac catheters
- ❏ B large area diathermy plates
- ❏ C battery-powered appliances
- ❏ D multiple earth paths
- ❏ E isolated (floating) power supply

3.76 Halothane vapour

- ❏ A concentration can be measured using a refractometer
- ❏ B is less dense than nitrous oxide
- ❏ C will absorb ultraviolet radiation
- ❏ D can be measured by infrared absorption
- ❏ E can be measured by changes in the elasticity of silicone rubber

3.77 Concerning the Mapleson classification of breathing systems

- ❑ A the Bain system is a Mapleson D system
- ❑ B all the systems are partial rebreathing systems
- ❑ C there are no valves in the Mapleson E system
- ❑ D the Mapleson A system is the most efficient for spontaneous ventilation
- ❑ E Humphrey designed a system incorporating the A, D and E systems into one breathing system

3.78 Nitrous oxide cylinders

- ❑ A are made of molybdenum steel
- ❑ B have a filling ratio of 0.67
- ❑ C the cylinder pressure is 137 bar
- ❑ D the cylinder pressure falls linearly with use
- ❑ E have a pin-index number of 3,6

3.79 The following are SI units

- ❑ A pascal
- ❑ B hertz
- ❑ C pounds per square inch
- ❑ D watt
- ❑ E joule

3.80 Cricoid pressure

- ❑ A was first described by Sellick
- ❑ B requires the application of a force of 440 newtons
- ❑ C is performed to prevent vomitus from entering the bronchial tree
- ❑ D must be applied at extubation as well as intubation
- ❑ E may make visualisation of the vocal cords more difficult

3.81 Pulse oximeters

- ❑ A may cause burns to the skin under the probe
- ❑ B are inaccurate in patients with pigmented skin
- ❑ C are inaccurate in the presence of haemoglobin F
- ❑ D are inaccurate in the presence of methaemoglobin
- ❑ E have a slower response time than transcutaneous oxygen electrodes

3.82 Regarding anaesthetic equipment

- ❏ A   a 14-G cannula can deliver a maximal flow rate of 280 ml/min
- ❏ B   a standard blood giving set has a filter of 150 μm diameter
- ❏ C   disposable endotracheal tubes are implant tested on mice
- ❏ D   the Fraser–Sweatman filling device for isoflurane is green
- ❏ E   the LMA should only be re-used 14 times

3.83 Regarding the gas laws

- ❏ A   Boyle's law states that at constant pressure the volume of a fixed mass of gas is inversely related to its temperature
- ❏ B   Avogadro's hypothesis states that the molar mass of a gas occupies 222.4 litres
- ❏ C   Charles' law states that at constant temperature the volume of a fixed mass of gas is inversely related to its pressure
- ❏ D $PV = kT$
- ❏ E   they all apply only to a gas at standard temperature and pressure

3.84 The Hagen–Poiseuille law states, assuming laminar flow, that

- ❏ A   the flow of liquid along a tube is inversely related to its length
- ❏ B   the flow is doubled for every doubling in diameter of the tube
- ❏ C   viscosity is not important
- ❏ D   density is not important
- ❏ E   the law only applies to Newtonian liquids

3.85 Capnography

- ❏ A   depends upon absorption of infrared light
- ❏ B   depends upon the presence of two or more different atoms in the molecule being measured
- ❏ C   the absorption spectra for carbon dioxide and nitrous oxide are widely separated
- ❏ D   may be inaccurate with very rapid respiratory rates
- ❏ E   reliably confirms correct placement of the endotracheal tube

3.86 Oxygen can be measured by

- ❏ A paramagnetic analyser
- ❏ B capnography
- ❏ C a fuel cell
- ❏ D cathode ray oscilloscope
- ❏ E pulse oximetry

3.87 Concerning the Mapleson E breathing system (Ayre's T-piece)

- ❏ A during spontaneous ventilation the fresh gas flow should be 2.5–3× the patient's minute volume
- ❏ B the volume of the corrugated tube must exceed the patient's tidal volume
- ❏ C Jackson-Rees modified the system by adding a closed bag to the end of the corrugated tube
- ❏ D scavenging from the Mapleson F system can be done easily
- ❏ E it should be used in children < 30 kg

3.88 The critical temperature

- ❏ A is the temperature above which that substance cannot be liquefied by pressure
- ❏ B of oxygen is –118°C
- ❏ C of nitrous oxide is 36.5°C
- ❏ D of carbon dioxide is 31°C
- ❏ E is the temperature below which that substance exists as liquid and vapour

3.89 The following are the correct pin-index numbers:

- ❏ A oxygen 2,5
- ❏ B air 1,5
- ❏ C nitrous oxide 3,5
- ❏ D helium 6,7
- ❏ E entonox no pin index

3.90 Nitrous oxide

- ❏   A   supports combustion
- ❏   B   was discovered by Joseph Priestley
- ❏   C   is supplied from pipelines at a pressure of 4 bar
- ❏   D   has a MAC of 1.05%
- ❏   E   has a boiling point of –88°C

MCQ Paper 3 – Answers

3.1   Answers: A D

The penicillins are bactericidal and act by inhibiting cell wall synthesis. Their principal side-effect is a hypersensitivity rash. The cephalosporins are bactericidal and interfere with the final stage of bacterial cell wall synthesis. Like the penicillins the principal side-effect of cephalosporins is a hypersensitivity rash. Ten per cent of patients with penicillin hypersensitivity will also be allergic to a cephalosporin.

The aminoglycosides act by binding to bacterial ribosomes leading to misreading of mRNA. The aminoglycosides are potentially ototoxic and nephrotoxic. Sulphonamides act as competitive antagonists of folic acid, which certain bacteria require.

Tetracyclines, like the aminoglycosides, bind to bacterial ribosomes.

3.2   Answers: D E

L-Dopa is the precursor of dopamine. L-Dopa crosses the blood–brain barrier but dopamine does not. L-Dopa is converted peripherally by the enzyme dopa-decarboxylase to dopamine. Patients are usually given, in addition to L-dopa, an L-dopa decarboxylase inhibitor to prevent this conversion as dopamine may cause arrhythmias or nausea.

3.3   Answer: C

Propofol is formulated in a white emulsion containing purified egg phosphatide, glycerol and soya bean oil. The pH of propofol is 10.

Propofol is metabolised mainly in the liver and conjugated to inactive products which are then excreted in the urine. Total body clearance is 1.5–2 l/min. Although propofol causes peripheral vasodilatation it has little effect on the coronary vasculature.

3.4   Answers: A B C D E

α2-Adrenoreceptor agonists, such as clonidine, act to reduce sympathetic outflow from the central nervous system. This results in bradycardia and hypotension. In addition these drugs are sedative and analgesic and reduce the requirement for other anaesthetic agents. They also cause a dry mouth and may cause Raynaud's phenomenon.

3.5 Answers: B C D E

The answer to this question lies in the two equations:
1. Blood pressure (BP) = cardiac output (CO) × total peripheral resistance (TPR)
2. CO = stroke volume (SV) × heart rate (HR).

TPR is controlled by vasoconstriction, produced by stimulation of α1-adrenoreceptors. These receptors are stimulated by the neurotransmitter noradrenaline released from nerve terminals.

Block of β receptors will cause a fall in heart rate and stroke volume thus leading to hypotension.

3.6 Answers: A C E

Tricyclic antidepressants act by inhibiting the re-uptake of noradrenaline into nerve terminals. In addition they have anticholinergic effects and this is why they are often associated with tachycardia, palpitations and arrhythmias, as well as dry mouth and constipation. Their onset of action may take several weeks, whilst the unwanted side-effects may occur much earlier.

3.7 Answers: A B C E

Ketamine is a phencyclidine derivative which acts at NMDA receptors. It is a racemic mixture, the + enantiomer being responsible for the useful effects such as analgesia and the – enantiomer being responsible for the side-effects. It is a sympathomimetic agent causing tachycardia, increased cardiac output and hypertension. It acts very slowly compared with other anaesthetic agents and it has active metabolites, such as nor-ketamine.

3.8 Answers: B C E

Most thiazide and loop diuretics lead to hypokalaemia. Amiloride and triamterene are potassium-sparing diuretics. Acetazolamide is a carbonic anhydrase inhibitor. Spironolactone is an aldosterone antagonist, and therefore is potassium sparing.

3.9 Answers: B C

β-blockers are negatively chronotropic and inotropic. Thus they reduce myocardial oxygen consumption and increase maximal exercise capacity. Some β-blockers are partial agonists and some have quinidine-like membrane stabilising effects. Whilst β-blockers may cause peripheral vaso-constriction, they have no effect on hepatic blood flow.

3.10 Answers: B E

Drugs which are highly ionised cannot cross the blood–brain barrier, whilst lipid-soluble drugs can. Equally drugs which are highly protein bound or of a large molecular weight do not cross readily. All of the anticholinesterases, except physostigmine, are highly ionised quaternary amines and therefore do not cross the blood–brain barrier. Hyoscine and atropine are both tertiary amines, less ionised, and thus able to cross. Glycopyrrolate is a quaternary amine. Morphine crosses the barrier because of its very high lipid solubility.

3.11 Answers: A D

Diazepam, as a benzodiazepine, acts within the central nervous system by stimulating inhibitory γ-aminobutyric acid receptors (GABA type A receptors). Onset of action is slower than that of thiopentone whilst the elimination half-life is prolonged, due mainly to the production of active metabolites such as temazepam, oxazepam and N-desmethyldiazepam, which has an elimination half-life of between 40 and 200 hours!

3.12 Answers: A B C D

Pharmacokinetics, the absorption, distribution, metabolism and excretion of drugs, may be described as what the body does to the drug. Pharmacodynamics, pharmacological effects at receptor level, may be described as what the drug does to the body. In zero-order kinetics a constant amount of drug is metabolised per unit of time.

This applies to alcohol which is metabolised by the enzyme alcohol dehy-drogenase. In first-order kinetics a constant percentage of drug is metabo-lised per unit of time. It is possible for kinetics to change from first to zero order, as can happen with phenytoin, for example.

The volume of distribution (V_d) is the apparent volume into which the drug is spread and depends on fat solubility to a large extent.

Drugs with a large V_d tend to be metabolised relatively slowly and so have long half-lives. Compartment models are used to describe the pharmacokinetics of drugs, although compartments do not refer to actual anatomical entities.

3.13 Answers: A B E

Tubocurarine, pancuronium and vecuronium are all partly excreted in bile and therefore in severe liver disease their action is potentiated. Gallamine is mainly excreted renally and its action is not significantly potentiated in liver disease. Atracurium is unique in that its metabolism and elimination are independent of either renal or liver function. It undergoes a pH-dependent spontaneous process termed Hoffman degradation and alkaline ester hydrolysis. Suxamethonium is metabolised by plasma cholinesterase, concentrations of which are much reduced in severe liver disease.

Neostigmine acts by competitively antagonising the action of the enzyme acetylcholinesterase, and it is unaffected by liver disease.

3.14 Answer: A

Phenytoin is extensively protein bound. Other anaesthetic drugs which are highly protein bound include the local anaesthetic agents and thiopentone.

3.15 Answers: B C

The size of the pupil is controlled by the autonomic nervous system.

Parasympathetic stimulation causes miosis, whilst dilatation of the pupil is caused by sympathetic stimulation. Thus neostigmine, by inhibiting the breakdown of acetylcholine, is parasympathomimetic and causes miosis. Opiates, such as codeine, stimulate the Edinger–Westphal nucleus of the oculomotor nerve, which is a purely parasympathetic nerve. It is by this mechanism that they cause miosis. Atenolol acts as a competitive antagonist at β-adrenoreceptors. The pupil is innervated by α-1 receptors, so β-blockers have no effect on the size of the pupil. Cocaine inhibits the re-uptake of noradrenaline at nerve endings and this sympathomimetic effect causes pupillary dilatation. Ganglion blockers cause mydriasis.

3.16 Answers: A C D

Plasma cholinesterase is responsible for the metabolism of a number of drugs including suxamethonium, mivacurium and the ester group of local anaesthetic agents, of which procaine is one.

3.17 Answer: D

Zero-order kinetics (saturation kinetics) occur when a drug is metabolised by an enzyme. This applies to alcohol which is metabolised by alcohol dehydrogenase. The quantity of alcohol metabolised per unit time is constant as the enzyme system is saturable. Although phenytoin may exhibit first- and zero-order kinetics, it only exhibits zero-order kinetics in excessive doses.

3.18 Answers: A B C

Sodium nitroprusside (SNP) is a vasodilator which acts via conversion to nitric oxide. The solution, once prepared, is unstable and must therefore be protected from light. Reflex tachycardia is marked with SNP. SNP may lead to an increase in intracranial pressure due to dilatation of cerebral vessels. SNP will lower pulmonary artery pressure.

3.19 Answers: A D E

The clearance of a drug (Cl) is the volume of plasma that is cleared of the drug in unit time. $Cl = V_d \times k$, where V_d is volume of distribution.

3.20 Answers: A B C D E

All of the drugs mentioned have a very long half-life. Diazepam has a half-life in excess of 200 hours due to its conversion to a number of active metabolites. Thiopentone undergoes metabolism according to zero-order kinetics so that only 10%–15% of the original dose of drug is eliminated every hour.

3.21 Answers: All false

The myocardium is supplied with oxygenated blood by the right and left coronary arteries. Venous drainage from the left ventricle passes via the coronary sinus to the right atrium.

Coronary blood flow occurs mainly in diastole and is therefore dependent upon diastolic blood pressure. In addition, as the length of diastole is dependent on heart rate, so is the coronary perfusion.

As β-blockade slows heart rate it leads to improved myocardial blood flow. Coronary blood flow is determined primarily by myocardial oxygen demand. Small changes in blood pressure in the healthy person have little effect on coronary blood flow due to autoregulation in the vascular bed.

3.22 Answers: B C D E

In starvation, body glycogen stores are exhausted within 24–48 hours and subsequent energy must be obtained from other sources.

Ketone bodies can be used by the brain but glucose is still essential. Hypokalaemia occurs and may be fatal.

3.23 Answers: A C E

The rate at which the alveolar concentration (F_A) of an anaesthetic agent approaches the inspired concentration (F_I) depends on:
- inspired concentration
- alveolar ventilation
- blood/gas solubility of the agent
- cardiac output.

The alveolar concentration of the agent rises more rapidly as the alveolar ventilation increases. The relation with cardiac output is inverse. The alveolar concentration of an agent that is relatively insoluble in blood will rise more rapidly than that of a soluble agent. The rate at which F_A approaches F_I is directly related to the inspired concentration of the agent.

3.24 Answers: B C D E

Metabolic acidosis is characterised by a reduced pH, reduced plasma bicarbonate and a base deficit. The normal compensatory mechanism is hyperventilation and a reduction in P_aCO_2, although the P_aCO_2 may be normal.

The normal plasma bicarbonate is 22–30 mmol/l. In acidosis this is reduced.

3.25 Answers: A D E

Active transport is the movement of a substance across a membrane against a concentration gradient. This requires expenditure of energy and is therefore affected by hypoxia and temperature. Active transport systems are characterised by maximal transport rates.

3.26 Answers: B C E

Iron is absorbed in the small intestine and transported in the plasma as transferrin. Iron is stored as ferritin. The amount of iron absorbed is determined by the amount of ferritin and by total iron binding capacity. Iron overload, haemosiderosis, may cause glucose intolerance.

3.27 Answers: A B E

Although both ventilation and perfusion are greater in the lower lung, the increase in blood flow is greater than the increase in ventilation and thus the V/Q is less in blood coming from the lower lung. This means that blood from the lower lung has a lower P_aO_2 and a higher P_aCO_2.

3.28 Answer: C

On changing from standing to supine the heart rate falls and the blood pressure increases. As a result there is decreased baroreceptor activity.

3.29 Answers: All false

Acetylcholine is the neurotransmitter at all autonomic ganglia.

3.30 Answer: A

During quiet inspiration the diaphragm and intercostal muscles are active but the accessory muscles such as sacrospinalis are not used.

Intrathoracic pressure decreases by 5–10 cmH$_2$O and alveolar volume increases by one-third.

3.31 Answers: B C E

Immediately after transection of the spinal cord so-called spinal shock occurs. This consists of hypotension due to loss of sympathetic tone, areflexia and loss of sensation below the level of cord transection.

3.32 Answers: C D E

Pain sensation is transmitted by fibres travelling in the spinothalamic tracts. It is vibration and joint position sense that are conveyed in the dorsal columns. The endorphins are endogenous opioid-like substances which are analgesic. The sensation of pain can be modified by strenuous exercise or by non-painful stimuli in the same area; this is how transcutaneous nerve stimulation (TENS) works.

3.33 Answers: D E

Gamma motor efferent fibres are found solely in striated skeletal muscle and are not present in the smooth muscle found in the uterus and vascular wall. Increased activity in these efferents leads to increased muscle tone and hyper-reflexia.

3.34 Answers: A C D

The ductus arteriosus is a connection between the pulmonary artery and aorta which is patent in the neonate and closes shortly after birth when the pulmonary vascular resistance drops. The ductus carries blood which has entered the right heart from the superior vena cava. This blood then passes from the pulmonary artery to the descending aorta. The foramen ovale is another temporary connection in the fetal heart, in this case between the atria. At birth the rise in left atrial pressure and drop in pulmonary vascular resistance lead to closure of the foramen ovale, although 10% of adults have a functionally patent foramen ovale.

3.35 Answers: A B C D E

Aldosterone is a mineralocorticoid steroid hormone produced by the zona glomerulosa of the adrenal cortex. It acts on the distal tubule of the kidney, promoting sodium reabsorption in exchange for potassium and hydrogen ions. The production of aldosterone is controlled by the renin–angiotensin system. Renin is produced by the juxtaglomerular apparatus of the afferent arteriole of the glomerulus. Its secretion is increased in response to hypo-volaemia, reduced renal blood flow and hyponatraemia. Renin acts on angiotensinogen, a plasma protein, converting it to angiotensin I, which in turn is converted to angiotensin II. Angiotensin II is an extremely potent vasoconstrictor and leads to the release of aldosterone. Aldosterone release is also stimulated by surgical stress, anxiety and haemorrhage. In addition hyponatraemia, hyperkalaemia and adrenocorticotrophic hormone (ACTH) all cause increased aldosterone release.

3.36 Answers: A B C E

Haemorrhage leads to increased sympathetic activity, with vasoconstriction and tachycardia. This helps to maintain cardiac output and keep vital organs such as the brain, kidneys and heart perfused. The reduced renal perfusion that results from haemorrhage activates the renin–angiotensin–aldosterone system and leads to increased release of antidiuretic hormone (ADH) from the posterior pituitary. This collective neurohumoral response leads to renal retention of sodium and water, restoring intravascular volume. In the longer term, haemorrhage will stimulate erythropoietin production by the kidney, which in turn stimulates the bone marrow to produce more red cells. The baroreceptors are stretch receptors located in the walls of the aortic arch and the carotid sinus. Haemorrhage leads to a reduction in baroreceptor activity. Afferent information from these receptors travels via the IX cranial nerve to the vasomotor centre in the medulla. Reduced afferent activity leads to increased efferent output from the vasomotor centre via the sympathetic nervous system. The chemoreceptors are either central or peripheral. The former respond to pH and P_aO_2 and are concerned with the control of respiration. The peripheral chemoreceptors, located in the aortic and carotid bodies, respond to hypoxaemia and hypoperfusion. Stimulation leads to increased sympathetic activity.

3.37 Answers: A B C E

The integrity of the baroreceptors and the autonomic nervous system can be tested by the Valsalva manoeuvre. The Valsalva manoeuvre is a forced expiration against a closed glottis. Initially this causes a transient rise in blood pressure as the rise in intrathoracic pressure expels a bolus of blood from the heart. The rise in intrathoracic pressure, however, reduces venous return and thus cardiac output and blood pressure drop. This is sensed by the baroreceptors which leads to increased sympathetic activity, vasoconstriction and tachycardia and a return of blood pressure towards normal. At the end of the Valsalva manoeuvre there is a transient rebound bradycardia and rise in blood pressure until the baroreceptors readjust. In patients with autonomic neuropathy, such as diabetics, there may be an abnormal response to the Valsalva manoeuvre.

3.38 Answers: A D

Potassium homeostasis is under the control of the hormone aldosterone. Potassium is excreted in very small amounts in health, it is filtered by the glomerulus and actively reabsorbed in the distal tubule. Postoperatively potassium excretion increases at least for the first few days.

3.39 Answers: A D E

There are three main clotting pathways: the intrinsic, extrinsic and common. The common pathway can be activated by either the extrinsic or intrinsic. The extrinsic pathway involves factor VII, whilst the intrinsic incorporates factors VIII, IX, XI and XII. The extrinsic path takes about 14 seconds, whilst the intrinsic is about twice as long. The common pathway is essentially the conversion of factor X to Xa. Factor Xa then converts prothrombin to thrombin, which in turn converts fibrinogen to fibrin. All the clotting factors are enzymes, many produced in the liver. Factors II, VII, IX and X are the vitamin-K-dependent factors.

3.40 Answers: B D E

Cerebrospinal fluid (CSF) is produced by the choroid plexus in the walls of the lateral ventricles at a rate of 0.4 ml/min. It is reabsorbed by the arachnoid villi. The volume of CSF is about 140 ml, about 10% of intracranial volume. The normal CSF pressure is 10–15 cmH$_2$O and varies with respiration and blood pressure.

3.41 Answers: A B C D

Both alcohol and mercury thermometers can be used to measure temperature. The Seebeck effect is employed in the thermocouple and resistance is used in both platinum resistance thermometers and thermistors.

3.42 Answers: All false

Boiling in water for 15 min at atmospheric pressure kills bacteria, but not spores. An autoclave pressure of 2–3 bar at 135°C for 3 min will kill all living organisms.

A 0.05% solution of chlorhexidine will sterilise an endotracheal tube in 30 min.

Ethylene oxide is effective against all organisms. At 55°C it takes about 2 hours, whilst at lower temperatures it takes up to 5 hours.

In all cases, however, aeration takes a further 7 days.

3.43 Answers: B D

The minimum alveolar concentration (MAC) is a concept first introduced by Eger and Merkel in 1963. MAC is the concentration of an anaesthetic agent that prevents the movement of 50% of the population to a standardised stimulus. It is measured at 1 atmosphere in fit, healthy male volunteers. It is an index of the potency of inhalational anaesthetic agents. The product of the oil/gas coefficient and MAC is, for most agents, a constant. MAC of an agent is given as a volume %; for example the MAC of nitrous oxide is 105%. MAC is affected by a host of factors including age, other drugs, pyrexia and atmospheric pressure.

3.44 Answer: B

The body plethysmograph is used to measure airway resistance.

3.45 Answers: All false

Basal metabolic rate for an average adult male is about 20 kJ/m^2 per h. It is measured using a spirometer. Basal metabolic rate is higher in children and is increased by anxiety and in thyrotoxicosis. Not all patients with a goitre are thyrotoxic, indeed many are either hypothyroid or euthyroid. Basal metabolic rate is lower in the tropics.

3.46 Answers: C D

About 60% of an average 70-kg male is total body water, ie 42 litres. Of this, two-thirds is intracellular fluid and one-third is extracellular fluid. Two-thirds of extracellular fluid is interstitial and one-third is plasma volume. Plasma volume can be measured using Evans' blue or radioactively labelled albumin. The extracellular fluid volume can be measured with inulin. Inulin is also used to measure glomerular filtration rate (GFR). Creatinine is also often used to measure GFR. *para*-Aminohippuric acid is used to measure renal plasma flow.

3.47 Answers: A C E

Oxygen rotameters are variable-orifice flowmeters. They consist of a bobbin in a cylinder and the scale along the side of the cylinder is non-linear. Each rotameter is calibrated for the specific gas it will carry, although in theory it is possible to use nitrous oxide with an oxygen rotameter. Rotameters may be affected by back pressure.

3.48 Answers: A B C D E

Pressure is defined as force per unit area. Pressure can be expressed as pascals (the SI unit of pressure), pounds per square inch (Imperial units) and bars.

A pascal is equal to 1 kg/s^2, which in turn can be expressed as a newton/m^2.

3.49 Answer: B

Oxygen and nitric oxide are attracted into a magnetic field; they are para-magnetic. This property is used in the paramagnetic analyser to measure the concentration of oxygen in a gas sample. These analysers are very accurate, sensitive and have a rapid response time.

3.50 Answers: A B C D E

The unit of electrical resistance is the ohm. The ohm is that resistance which will allow one ampere of current to flow under the influence of a potential of one volt. Ohm's law states that resistance (R) = potential (V)/current (I). A rise in temperature increases the resistance of a wire resistor. Resistance rises as the tension or length of a wire increases.

3.51 Answers: A C D

Viscosity affects laminar flow according to the Hagen–Poiseuille formula. The viscosity of a liquid is inversely related to the temperature. With turbulent flow, density becomes the important factor. Heliox (oxygen/helium) is less dense than oxygen/nitrous oxide and is used to relieve inspiratory stridor where turbulent flow is a problem.

3.52 Answer: C

Surface tension is due to attraction between molecules in a liquid. It is measured in either newtons/m or dynes/cm. It is independent of either temperature or viscosity. It leads to a mercury manometer under-reading.

3.53 Answers: A D

Boyle's law states that at constant temperature the volume of a fixed mass of gas varies inversely with the absolute pressure. A plot of P versus V is a rectangular hyperbola. One mole of any gas at standard temperature and pressure occupies 22.4 litres.

3.54 Answers: A D

Mercury thermometers have a very slow response time, whereas platinum resistance thermometer probes have a very rapid response time. Thermistors can become unreliable if exposed to high temperatures.

3.55 Answers: A B C D

There are several ways of humidifying inspired gases including the nose! The artificial nose or heat and moisture exchanger (HME) is most commonly used in clinical practice. Other methods that have been employed include passage of gas through a cold or hot water bath or the use of nebulisers, some of which work by using the Bernoulli effect.

3.56 Answers: C D E

The physical properties of nitrous oxide are:
Blood/gas solubility 0.47
MAC value of 105%
Filling ratio of 0.75
Critical temperature of 36.5°C
Critical pressure of 72.6 bar
Boiling point of –88°C

3.57 Answer: D

To measure central venous pressure (CVP) a catheter is inserted via usually the subclavian or internal jugular vein. When a reading is taken the patient should be lying flat and, if connected to a ventilator, it should be taken at the end of expiration. The zero of the scale is the midaxillary line. The catheters tend to be long and narrow.

3.58 Answers: A B C

Henry's law states that at a particular temperature the amount of a given gas dissolved in a given liquid is directly proportional to the partial pressure of the gas in equilibrium with the liquid.

3.59 Answer: All false.

Spirometry only measures FEV_1 and FEV.

3.60 Answers: A B D E

In circle systems the vaporiser may be located within the circle (VIC) or outside the circle (VOC). With a VIC, at low flows the vapour concentration will be higher than that dialled up. With a VOC the vapour concentration will be lower than that dialled up. It is thus important to monitor gas concentrations in a circle system.

3.61 Answer: B

One atmosphere is equivalent to –1 bar, 101.3 kPa, 760 mmHg, 1000 cmH$_2$O, 14.7 Psi and 750 torr.

3.62 Answer: C

The intra-aortic balloon pump (IABP) is inserted via the femoral artery and positioned in the descending aorta, just distal to the left subclavian artery. Inflation is synchronised to the patient's ECG. It is inflated with 50 ml of helium at the onset of diastole. This results in increased aortic diastolic pressure, improved coronary perfusion and improved myocardial oxygen delivery. Deflation occurs just prior to systole thus decreasing left ventricular afterload and left ventricular work.

3.63 Answers: A D E

Pacemakers may be affected by anaesthetic drugs, MRI scanners, shivering, diathermy and many other factors. Bipolar diathermy is safer than unipolar and MRI scanning is absolutely contraindicated in patients with a pacemaker. A demand pacemaker can readily be converted to a fixed rate pacemaker by placing a magnet over it. Pacemakers are becoming increasingly more sophisticated and the manufacturers should be consulted about the effect of placing a magnet over the pacemaker before doing so. The pacemaker function should also be checked by a specialist technician postoperatively if a magnet is used, because the magnet can produce a permanent change in programming in some models.

3.64 Answers: A B C D

Entonox is the trade name for a 50:50 mixture of oxygen and nitrous oxide. It can be administered by registered midwives and is used for analgesia in labour. It is stored at a pressure of 137 bar and has a pseudocritical temperature of ~ –7°C (stated to be between –5.5°C and –8°C). The pseudocritical temperature is the temperature at which the gases separate out. This is important because there is a risk of delivering a hypoxic mixture if the cylinder is stored at a low temperature. Because of the Poynting effect the presence of oxygen reduces the critical temperature of nitrous oxide and at 137 bar the two gases dissolve in each other. Nitrous oxide inhibits the enzyme methionine synthetase and by this mechanism may, after prolonged exposure, cause megaloblastic anaemia.

3.65 Answers: A B C D E

The standard Tuohy needle is 16 G, has Lees lines every 1 cm and is 10 cm in length. At its tip is the Huber point and there may be Macintosh wings that can be attached to the needle. The bacterial filter has pores of 22 μm diameter. The epidural space may be located by the loss of resistance to air or saline technique or by the hanging drop method.

3.66 Answers: B D

In an exponential process after one time constant the value will have fallen to 37% of its original and after three time constants 95% of the process is complete.

3.67 Answer: C

Helium is stored as a gas at room temperature in brown cylinders at a pressure of 137 bar. It has a similar viscosity to oxygen but is far less dense. Its low density causes the voice changes seen when it is inhaled and makes it useful in upper airway obstruction such as stridor due to laryngeal obstruction. It is however of no value in treating bronchospasm. It does not support combustion nor is it narcotic at high pressure.

3.68 Answers: A B D

The Wright's respirometer is a turbine which measures gas volume, such as tidal or minute volume. It under reads at <1 l/min and is affected by moisture which causes the pointer to stick. The pneumotachograph measures flow rate such as peak flow and is affected by gas viscosity.

3.69 Answers: B C D E

Peak flow is measured by the pneumotachograph. It has a normal diurnal variation and is reduced in an acute attack of asthma. The peak flow is usually used to monitor the response to therapy in an asthmatic. The measurement of peak flow is very dependent on effort.

3.70 Answers: C E

The Severinghaus electrode is used to measure the tension of carbon dioxide in blood: the P_aCO_2. In fact, it is the concentration of hydrogen ions (the pH) that is actually measured but this is directly related to P_aCO_2. The CO_2 in blood diffuses across a semipermeable membrane and reacts with water to produce carbonic acid which then dissociates to hydrogen and bicarbonate ions. This reaction takes place at the pH-sensitive glass electrode, which is bathed in bicarbonate ions. The pH is measured and from that the P_aCO_2 is calculated.

3.71 Answer: E

Soda lime is used to absorb CO_2 in anaesthetic breathing systems.

It contains approximately 90% calcium hydroxide. Sodium hydroxide (5%) and potassium hydroxide (1%) are present as catalysts for the reaction between soda lime and CO_2. An indicator dye is present to show when the soda lime is exhausted. The reaction is exothermic and produces heat. Soda lime is compatible with all the currently used volatile agents, although sevoflurane is degraded to compound A at high temperatures. Although nephrotoxic in rats there is no evidence that compound A is harmful to humans. Carboxyhaemoglobinaemia may occur when certain volatile agents react with dried out soda lime.

3.72 Answers: A B C D E

All of the options are potential complications of the siting of an arterial line.

3.73 Answers: A B C D

Thromboelastography is used to assess coagulation status. It is particularly useful in providing information on platelet function and fibrinolysis, neither of which is provided by the laboratory estimation of PT, aPTT and platelet count. It takes, however, no longer to run than the laboratory tests. It is exquisitely sensitive to heparin, although any heparin effect can be blocked by adding heparinase reagent to the blood sample before running the TEG.

The use of blood products such as FFP and platelets and the need for, for example, aprotinin or tranexamic acid can be ascertained from the TEG.

3.74 Answers: A B C E

The transoesophageal Doppler probe employs high-frequency sound waves. It can be used to assess cardiac output, segmental wall motion abnormalities and volaemic status. It is very sensitive to the presence of pulmonary emboli and can also be used to view heart valve anatomy.

3.75 Answers: C E

Microshock is the term used to describe the delivery of very small currents (100–150 μA) directly to the myocardium, where they may cause ventricular fibrillation. Microshock requires the presence of a faulty intracardiac catheter (eg CVP line or pacemaker electrode) touching the wall of the heart along which current can flow.

Whilst 5% dextrose will not conduct current, saline certainly will.

The severity of microshock is inversely related to current frequency so risk is greatest at low frequencies such as mains frequency.

3.76 Answers: A C D E

Halothane will absorb ultraviolet and infrared radiation and will cause a change in the elasticity of silicone rubber. Halothane concentration can also be determined by a refractometer.

Halothane has a molecular weight of 197 Da: that of nitrous oxide is 44 Da.

3.77 Answers: A C D E

In 1954, Mapleson devised a classification for the breathing systems in use. They were labelled A to E; the A is the Magill (or Lack coaxial version). It is the most efficient for spontaneous ventilation. The D system is the Bain and is the most efficient for controlled ventilation.

The E is the Ayre's T-piece and is the paediatric system used for children weighing less than 20 kg. This system was modified by Jackson-Rees who added an open-ended bag; this became the F system.

3.78 Answers: A B

Nitrous oxide is stored in French blue cylinders made of molybdenum steel. The pressure at 20°C is 54 bar; oxygen is stored at 137 bar. Because nitrous oxide is stored as a liquid it is present as a saturated vapour and the pressure in the cylinder only begins to fall once all the liquid has evaporated through use. The filling ratio is 0.67 and the critical temperature 36.5°C. The pin-index number for cyclopropane was 3,6; that for nitrous oxide is 3,5.

3.79 Answers: A B D E

3.80 Answers: A E

Sellick's manoeuvre, or the application of cricoid pressure, is designed to prevent the passive regurgitation of acidic gastric contents. It requires the application of a force of 44 newtons. It is performed by compressing the oesophagus between the cricoid cartilage and the vertebral body of C6; either as a one- or two-handed technique. It should not be applied if vomiting occurs as it may cause rupture of the oesophagus. Although it is sometimes used to aid visualisation of the cords it may have the opposite effect. Although pressure is sometimes applied over the larynx to help visualisation of the larynx, this is not the same as the technique used to apply cricoid pressure for prevention of passive regurgitation.

3.81 Answer: D

Pulse oximeters do not cause burns. They are inaccurate in the presence of both methaemoglobin and carboxyhaemoglobin but are unaffected by pigmented skin or the presence of fetal haemoglobin F.

3.82 Answers: A B

Disposable endotracheal tubes are implant tested on rabbits. The LMA may be re-used up to 50 times. The Fraser-Sweatman keyed filling devices are colour coded and the colour for isoflurane is purple.

3.83 Answer: D

The gas laws are as follows:
1. Boyle's law states that at constant temperature the volume of a gas is inversely proportional to the pressure.
2. Charles' law states that at constant pressure the volume of a gas is directly proportional to the temperature.
3. Gay-Lussac's law states that at constant volume the pressure of a gas is directly proportional to the temperature.
This leads to the combined (Universal) gas law: $PV = kT$, where k is a constant. Although not a gas law, Avogadro's hypothesis states that the

gram molecular weight of a gas occupies 22.4 litres at standard temperature and pressure (STP).

3.84 Answers: A D E

The Hagen–Poiseuille formula relates to laminar flow of Newtonian fluids through a tube. The formula shows that flow is inversely related to viscosity; density is a factor only in turbulent, non-laminar flow. Flow increases fourfold for every doubling of diameter of the tube.

3.85 Answers: A B D E

Capnography, or the measurement of end-tidal CO_2, uses the principle of infrared absorption spectrophotometry. Infrared light is absorbed by any gas with two or more different atoms in the molecule, hence nitrous oxide will also absorb it. This is known as the Luft principle. The absorption spectra for infrared light for carbon dioxide and nitrous oxide are very close. The presence of a capnograph waveform reliably confirms the correct placement of an endotracheal tube.

3.86 Answers: A C

Oxygen may be measured by fuel cell, mass spectrometer, paramagnetic analyser, chemically or polarographically. As oxygen has unpaired electrons it is attracted to a magnetic field (ie it is paramagnetic). Once in a magnetic field oxygen molecules become agitated, resulting in a change in pressure proportional to the oxygen concentration. This is detected by a transducer and converted into a displayed signal.

3.87 Answers: A B

The Mapleson E breathing system takes its name from its inventor Dr Philip Ayre who was a neuroanaesthetist in Newcastle, and designed it in 1937. It was later modified by Dr Jackson-Rees, an anaesthetist in Liverpool. He added an open-ended bag to Ayre's T-piece.

For efficient spontaneous respiration the fresh gas flow needs to be 2–3 times the patient's minute volume and, in addition, the volume of the corrugated tubing must exceed the patient's tidal volume. It should be used in children of 20 kg or less. Although scavenging from the system is possible, it is not particularly easy.

3.88 Answers: A B C D E

The critical temperature is the temperature above which a gas cannot be liquefied by pressure.

3.89 Answers: A B C

The pin-index system was designed to prevent the wrong gas cylinder being attached to an anaesthetic machine. One or more pins project from the yoke and these fit into holes on the cylinder.

The configuration of the pins is specific to each gas.
Oxygen is 2,5
Air 1,5
Nitrous oxide 3,5
Helium no pin
Entonox a single pin position 7.

3.90 Answers: A B C E

Nitrous oxide was discovered by Joseph Priestley in 1772 and its anaesthetic properties were first suggested in 1799 by another Englishman, Sir Humphrey Davy. It was first used as an anaesthetic in 1844; just 21 months before the first use of ether. It is a sweet-smelling, non-irritant gas which though not explosive will support combustion. It has a boiling point of −88°C, a critical temperature of 36.5°C and a critical pressure of 72.6 bar. Its MAC value is 105%. It is supplied from pipelines at a pressure of 4 bar or from cylinders, stored at a pressure of 54 bar.

OSCE 1 – Questions

QUESTION 1

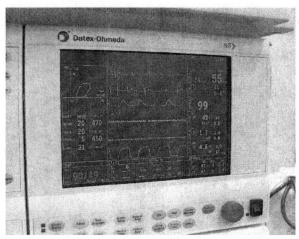

(a) What is Einthoven's law and how does this relate to the recording of any ECG? (3 marks)

(b) Mark on the diagram

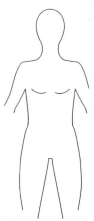

the position of the three leads (red, yellow and green) in the CM5 position. (3 marks)

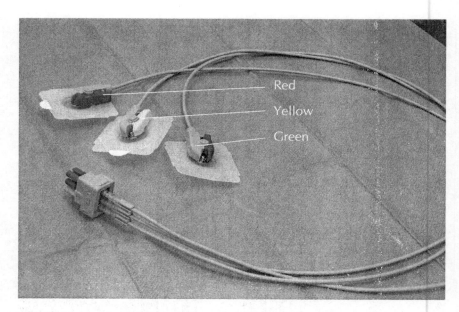

(c) What colour leads are most important for generating the following readings? (3 marks)

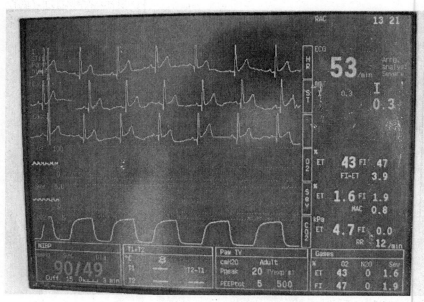

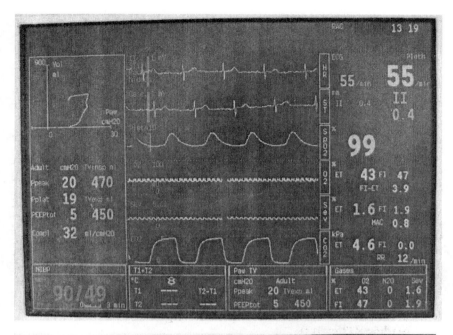

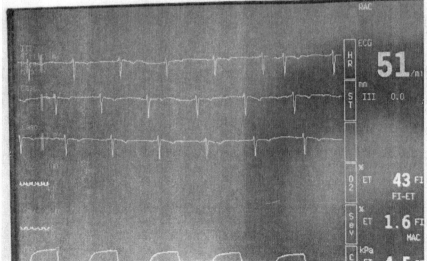

(d) What additional lead is required to calculate aVR? (1 mark)

(e) How is the recording for aVR, aVF and aVL calculated? (3 marks)

(f)   Write a description of the position of the leads V1 to V6 in the 12-lead ECG. (3 marks)

(g)   How many physical leads are required for the 12-lead ECG? (1 mark)

(h)   What is the purpose of the right lower limb lead in the 12-lead ECG? (1 mark)

(i)   What is the standard speed for a 12-lead ECG? (1 mark)

(j)   What is the standard calibration for a 12-lead ECG? (1 mark)

QUESTION 2

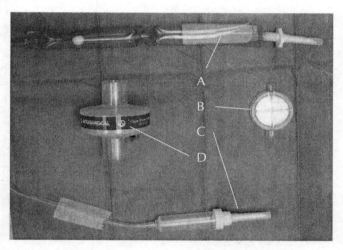

(a)   What are these four filters? (4 marks)

Answer the following True/False questions (1 mark each, no negative marking)

(b)   Filter B is likely to have a pore size of 20–40 μm.

(c)   Filter C is likely to have a pore size of 0.2 μm.

(d)   Filter A is effective at removing bacteria.

(e)   Filter C is effective at removing viral matter.

(f)   Filter D is made of a hydrophobic material.

(g)   Filter D when first used has a resistance of 10 cmH$_2$O.

(h)   The more filter B is used for the product it is designed for, the less efficient it becomes and should be changed every couple of hours.

(i)   The effectiveness of filter D is affected by anaesthetic gases.

(j)   Filter C could be used to transfuse blood in an emergency.

(k)   Both A and D should be changed every 24 h.
(l)   Filter D can achieve a relative humidity of up to 70%.
(m)   If an ultrasonic nebuliser is used in conjunction with D, on the circuit side, a much higher humidity can be achieved.
(n)   The function of A relies on electrostatic forces.
(o)   Filter B helps protect against bacterial contamination.
(p)   Filter A contains a Luer lock.
(q)   All filters are designed for reuse.

QUESTION 3

A woman with a mechanical heart valve presents to you for emergency surgery for a life-threatening lower GI bleed.

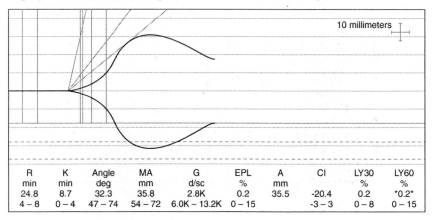

R min	K min	Angle deg	MA mm	G d/sc	EPL %	A mm	CI	LY30 %	LY60 %
24.8	8.7	32.3	35.8	2.8K	0.2	35.5	-20.4	0.2	*0.2*
4 – 8	0 – 4	47 – 74	54 – 72	6.0K – 13.2K	0 – 15		-3 – 3	0 – 8	0 – 15

INR	4.5
ACT	250 s
PTT	65 s
aPTT	2.5× normal
TT	25 s
Fibrinogen	0.9 g/l

Answer the following True/False questions (1 mark each, no negative marking)

(a)   The INR is appropriate for a patient with a mechanical valve.
(b)   The aPTT value and the ACT value both suggest that the patient has received heparin.

(c)   If the patient is pregnant, not bleeding but has a mechanical heart valve, the ideal aPTT is 2.5× normal.

(d)   The increased thrombin time is not surprising given the value for fibrinogen.

(e)   It is possible that her raised INR is the result of liver disease.

(f)   The determination of an INR involves the use of Manchester comparative reagent.

(g)   INR stands for International Normalised Reaction.

(h)   Protamine and heparin react as an acid and base.

(i)   In excess, protamine has an anticoagulant effect.

(j)   It would not be appropriate to give the patient fresh frozen plasma and cryoprecipitate.

(k)   Vitamin K would help correct the INR if the patient is on warfarin.

(l)   The final common pathway in the coagulation cascade involves factors I, II, V, XIII.

(m)   Aspirin will decrease the numbers of platelets in this patient.

(n)   Tranexamic acid acts as a substrate for plasmin.

(o)   Aprotinin, like tranexamic acid, helps prevent the breakdown of plasmin.

(p)   Dipyridamole inhibits the platelets' ability to release adenosine diphosphate.

(q)   This trace has come from a thromboelastograph.

(r)   The increased length of R could indicate a heparin effect.

(s)   The reduction in maximum amplitude indicates clot breakdown.

(t)   The reduction in maximum amplitude may be decreased by the use of tranexamic acid.

QUESTION 4

(a) Label the following diagram. (10 marks)

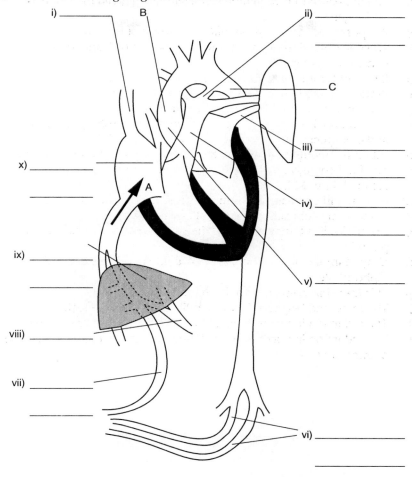

i) _____
B
ii) _____
_____
C
iii) _____
x) _____
_____
A
iv) _____
ix) _____
_____
v) _____
viii) _____
vii) _____
_____
vi) _____
_____

(b) Continue drawing the course of the majority of blood flow marked with arrow A. (3 marks)

(c) What is different about blood leaving the artery at point B compared to point C? (2 marks)

(d) Why is this important in the development of the fetus? (2 marks)

(e) What three physical changes have occurred to the circulation of the fetus by 3 months? (3 marks)

QUESTION 5

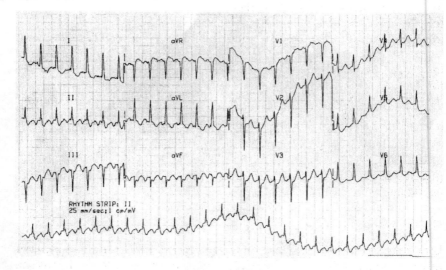

(a) What arrhythmia is shown? (2 marks)
(b) What are the diagnostic features of this on this ECG? (4 marks)
(c) How does this differ from other tachyarrythmias? (3 marks)
(d) What are the possible aetiologies? (4 marks)
(e) How would you treat this? (5 marks)
(f) Is anticoagulation required? (1 mark)
(g) What else does the ECG show? (1 mark)

QUESTION 6

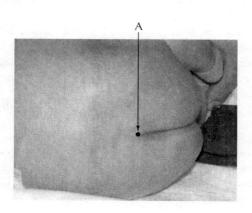

(a) What is marked by point A? (1 mark)
(b) What covers point A? (2 marks)
(c) What is contained in the canal beneath A? (4 marks)
(d) What two points form an equilateral triangle with A and are used in its location? (1 mark)
(e) Where is the dural sac likely to end in a 5-year-old? (1 mark)
(f) Where may the dural sac descend to in a newborn? (1 mark)
(g) What is the maximum volume of 0.25% bupivacaine a 20-kg child can have? (1 mark)
(h) What volume of bupivacaine is sufficient to perform mid thoracic surgery? What must be adjusted? (1 mark)
(i) How would you perform a caudal anaesthetic? (4 marks)
(j) What needs to be confirmed before the child is discharged? (2 marks)
(k) How does the sacral hiatus form? (2 marks)

QUESTION 7

For the next question you are faced with an obstetric woman who estimates her gestational period at 34 weeks. You have been asked to see her as she has problems with her blood pressure and is in the early stages of labour. Carry out an examination of the airway, abdominal and cardiovascular systems on this lady. When you have completed this you will be asked some questions by the examiner.

(a) Describe the sequence of actions that you would perform in assessing this lady. (In the exam you will be expected to perform the examination!) (15 marks)
(b) Would a creatinine of 95 µmol/l be considered normal? (1 mark)
(c) Is the fundal height of a lady of 24 weeks' gestation palpable at the level of the umbilicus? (1 mark)
(d) In late pregnancy can the functional residual capacity (FRC) of the pregnant woman improve? (1 mark)
(e) Is a PCO_2 of 4 kPa entirely normal in pregnancy? (1 mark)
(f) Is a decrease in diastolic blood pressure caused by increased levels of progesterone? (1 mark)

QUESTION 8

(a) Describe the anatomy of the right subclavian vein. (5 marks)
(b) Describe how you would perform cannulation of this vessel. (12 marks)
(c) What are the potential immediate complications of the procedure? (3 marks)

QUESTION 9

(a)   Name the following spinal tracts and structures that are pointed to in the diagram. (14 marks)

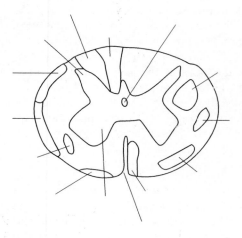

(b)   Describe the arterial supply to the spinal cord. (3 marks)

(c)   What clinical effect would the destruction of the ascending posterior columns and ascending spinocerebellar tracts have? (2 marks)

(d)   Describe the course of the lateral spinothalamic tract. (2 marks)

QUESTION 10

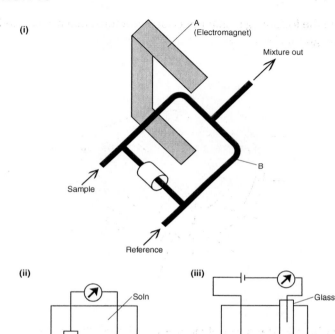

(a) Which one of these pictures shows a polarographic oxygen analyser? (1 mark)
(b) What makes up the anode? (2 marks)
(c) What constitutes the cathode? (1 mark)
(d) What does the solution contain? (1 mark)
(e) What covers the end of the cathode, and what characteristic does it have? (3 marks)
(f) Why is there a battery? (1 mark)
(g) What reaction occurs at the cathode? (4 marks)
(h) What reaction occurs at the anode? (4 marks)
(i) How is it calibrated? (2 marks)
(j) At what temperature is the sample measured? (1 mark)

QUESTION 11

History station
A Jehovah's Witness presents for a left mastectomy for a carcinoma. Take a history from her.

(a)   Discuss her presenting condition and its implications. What information do you need? (10 marks)
(b)   What issues surround her beliefs as a Jehovah's Witness, and what should you establish from her? (5 marks)
(c)   She tells you she has recently had haematuria; what do you need to find out about this? (5 marks)

QUESTION 12

'Sim' man
Drugs have just been given for a rapid sequence induction of a 20-year-old with a history of severe reflux having an arthroscopy.
You try to intubate the patient but he has severe masseter spasm.

(a)   Describe what you would do first. (2 marks)
(b)   You are unable to ventilate the patient. Describe what you would now do. State what sizes of the following equipment you require: a cannula, a syringe, an endotracheal tube and an Ambu bag. (6 marks)

Following this, a formal tracheostomy is established. However, the patient's end-tidal CO_2 continues to rise despite adequate ventilation and his temperature climbs to 42°C.

(c)   What is the presumptive diagnosis? (1 mark)
(d)   Describe your initial management. (11 marks)

QUESTION 13

(a)   Explain to a new ODP how you would perform a rapid sequence induction and how this would involve them. (15 marks)
(b)   Are there any circumstances in which cricoid pressure should be released prematurely? (2 marks)
(c)   In the event of failure to secure the airway, what is the role of the ODP? (3 marks)

QUESTION 14

(a) What general mechanisms of nerve injury can occur with anaesthesia and surgery? (6 marks)

(b) Are there any general risk factors for perioperative neuropraxias? (4 marks)

(c) What nerves are vulnerable in the following pictures? What are the clinical consequences of each of the nerve lesions? (8 marks)

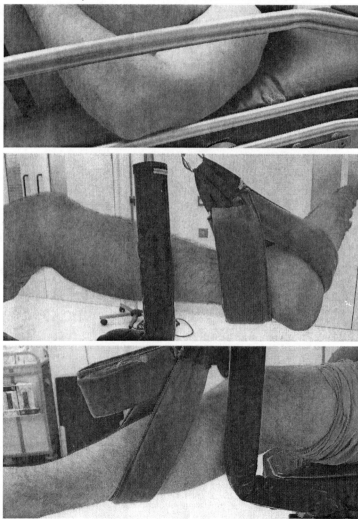

(d)　What might cause and what are the clinical consequences of an obturator nerve palsy or injury? (2 marks)

QUESTION 15

Answer the following questions

(a)　Where does the word capnograph come from? (1 mark)

(b)　At which point in the infrared spectrum does carbon dioxide have its greatest absorption? (1 mark)

(c)　If nitrous oxide is used, does this have the potential to result in a higher or lower reading than the actual carbon dioxide present? (1 mark)

(d)　Label the diagram below representing the various parts of the capnograph. Where is the gas flow coming from between B + C and C + D? Can this trace be used in lieu of Fowler's method? (4 marks)

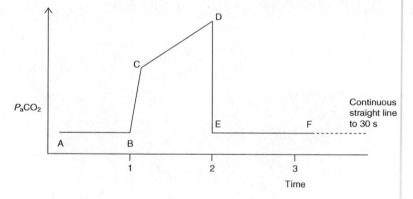

(e)　Does inspiration begin at point A? (1 mark)

(f)　Is expiration occurring at point B? (1 mark)

(g)　Does AB represent the inspiratory time? (1 mark)

(h)　Is CD normal? (1 mark)

(i)　Does CD represent abnormal alveolar mixing? (1 mark)

(j)　Could CD result from marked bronchospasm? (1 mark)

(k)　Under what conditions is your expired CO_2 greater than your alveolar CO_2 by 2 kPa? (1 mark)

(l)　Does EF represent air embolism? (1 mark)

(m)　Could EF be the result of breath holding? (1 mark)

(n)　Does cerebral hypoxia occur immediately? (1 mark)

(o)   Should surgery be stopped after EF has occurred? (1 mark)

The second trace is obtained after the patient is reintubated

(p)   What is this pattern consistent with? (2 marks)

QUESTION 16

You are presented with information from the intensive care records of a lady admitted 24 hours ago. She is 65 years old with a fluctuating level of consciousness and low urine output. She has a pulmonary artery catheter in situ.

Answer the questions based on the following information.

Temp	42°C	K$^+$	6.0 mmol/l
BP	80/40 mmHg	Cl$^-$	111 mmol/l
HR	110 bpm	HCO$_3^-$	10 mmol/l
CO	13 l/min	pH	7.2
SVR	700 dyne s/cm^5	P_aO_2	20 kPa (on F_iO_2 of 1.0)
PCWP	15 cmH$_2$O	P_aCO_2	5.0 kPa
PAP	32/14 mmHg	BE	−20 mmol/l
CVP	12 cmH$_2$O	S_aO_2	98%
Na$^+$	140 mmol/l	Lactate	3 mmol/l

(a) Is the tachycardia likely to be pain related? (1 mark)
(b) Is the SVR normal? (1 mark)
(c) Should you withhold antibiotic therapy until blood cultures have returned? (1 mark)
(d) Could this picture be explained by sepsis? (1 mark)
(e) What is the definition of sepsis? (3 marks)
(f) Could this be myocardial dysfunction? (1 mark)
(g) Would it be inappropriate to give a fluid bolus, given the already high CVP? (1 mark)
(h) Should the patient be treated with noradrenaline? (1 mark)
(i) Is adrenaline contraindicated if there is no urine output? (1 mark)
(j) Is the pulmonary capillary wedge pressure at the upper end of normal? (1 mark)
(k) What does the pulmonary capillary wedge pressure represent? Is it a more accurate measure of filling than CVP? (1 mark)
(l) Could the high pulmonary artery pressure be caused by a high pulmonary vascular resistance? (1 mark)
(m) What are the complications of a pulmonary artery catheter? (4 marks)
(n) There is an arterial alveolar gradient of greater than 60 kPa – does this make a diagnosis of ARDS possible? (1 mark)
(o) Could a low APACHE score be used as a basis for withdrawing treatment? (1 mark)

QUESTION 17

Consider the following data series:

3,4,6,6,7,2,4,5,1,6

(a) In this series, calculate values for the mean, median and mode. (3 marks)
(b) What are the following types of data: subarachnoid classification, blood pressure, and penile length? (3 marks)
(c) How are these data distributed? (1 mark)

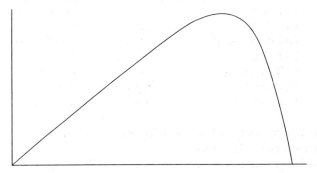

(d) How are the data distributed and what are their statistical characteristics? (6 marks)

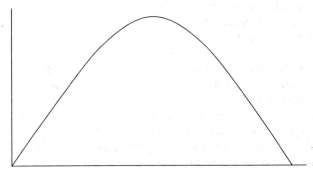

(e) What test could be used to determine whether there is a statistical difference in average height between the inhabitants of two continents? (2 marks)

(f)   If 20 papers are in the *BMJ* with a probability value of $p = 0.05$, how many results will have occurred by complete chance? (1 mark)

(g)   What is a type I (α) error? (1 mark)

(h)   What is a type II (β) error? (1 mark)

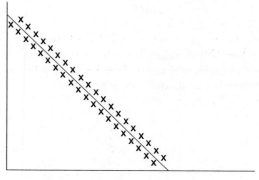

(i)   What is the correlation between the findings of height and money spent on health care? (2 marks)

OSCE 1 – Answers

ANSWER 1

(a) Einthoven's Law states that if the values for any two points of a triangle are known the third can be calculated. Therefore, in relation to an ECG only two leads are actually required to calculate the vector of the third.

(b)

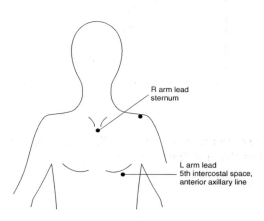

R arm lead
sternum

L arm lead
5th intercostal space,
anterior axillary line

(c) Lead I – red (right arm) and yellow (left arm)
Lead II – red and green (left leg or hip)
Lead III – yellow and green.

(d) No additional lead is required as aVR is calculated from leads I and II (see below).

(e) Connecting the three electrodes of the standard limb leads to a common central terminal allows a zero potential to be obtained. Taking this theoretical 'common electrode' and comparing it to the limb leads allows the potential differences to be measured. These are relatively small in size and so are electronically augmented (hence the 'a' in their notation).

(f) V1 – 4th intercostal space just to the right of the sternum
V2 – 4th intercostal space just to the left of the sternum
V3 – midway between V2 and V4
V4 – 5th intercostal space in the midclavicular line

V5 – same level as V4 on the anterior axillary line
V6 – 5th intercostal space, mid axillary line.
(g) Ten leads are required.
(h) It is used to act as a differential filter to reduce background noise. It is sometimes referred to as the 'Common mode reject' lead.
(i) The standard speed for an ECG is 25 mm/s.
(j) The standard calibration for an ECG is 10 mm/mV.

ANSWER 2

(a) A – Blood giving set filter
   B – Epidural filter
   C – Standard IV giving set filter
   D – Heat Moisture Exchanger (HME).
(b) *True* This is the standard range for a blood filter.
(c) *True* Filter C does have a filter size of 0.2 µm, much smaller than the blood filter.
(d) *True* Filter A is effective at removing bacteria, viruses and foreign bodies such as glass particles.
(e) *True* At a size of 0.2 µm it is effective at removing viral matter.
(f) *True* It is made of a hydrophobic material.
(g) *False* The resistance after many hours should only reach 3–4 cmH_2O.
(h) *False* This type of blood filter (depth) actually becomes more efficient through use. However, although it becomes more efficient at removing particulate matter, it has an effect on the flow characteristics and in times of high volume blood loss and replacement it may need to be replaced more often.
(i) *False* It is unaffected by anaesthetic gases.
(j) *False* The filter size is too small and would clog.
(k) *True* Both epidural filters and HMEs should be changed at least every 24 h.
(l) *True* This can be achieved by an HME.
(m) *False* The HME will become waterlogged and inefficient.
(n) *False* It works solely on mesh size.
(o) *False* The filter is not small enough and this is why bacterial infection is a complication of blood transfusion.
(p) *True* It has been argued that there should be an epidural-specific connection to prevent inadvertent intravenous administration of long-acting and potentially cardiotoxic local anaesthetics.
(q) *False* All filters are single use.

ANSWER 3

(a) *True* Although this is the upper range of anticoagulation required for a mechanical valve.

(b) *True* The raised aPPT and ACT both suggest the use of heparin.

(c) *False* For a pregnant woman aPPT range should be 1.5–2× normal.

(d) *True* Hypofibrinogenaemia will cause a prolonged thrombin time.

(e) *True* Liver disease can cause a raised INR.

(f) *True* INR or international normalised *ratio* uses a standard reagent to calculate the prothrombin time called the Manchester comparative reagent.

(g) *False* See (f).

(h) *True* This is the nature of the reaction by which protamine reverses the effects of heparin.

(i) *True* Excess protamine does act as an anticoagulant by activating thrombin receptors on platelets causing partial activation and thereby impeding platelet aggregation.

(j) *False* The coagulation results suggest both are needed.

(k) *True*

(l) *True*

(m) *False* It will not affect platelet numbers, only their function.

(n) *True* This is how it works.

(o) *False* They both prevent the breakdown of fibrin.

(p) *False* This is how aspirin works.

(q) *True*

(r) *True* R denotes the speed of clot formation and is lengthened by heparin and a reduction in clotting factors. Use of a heparinase-treated sample will reveal any systemic or contaminant heparin effect.

(s) *True* A TEG measures speed and strength of clot formation; an early decrease in maximum amplitude indicates clot lysis.

(t) *True* Tranexamic acid will reduce clot lysis by inhibiting plasmin.

ANSWER 4

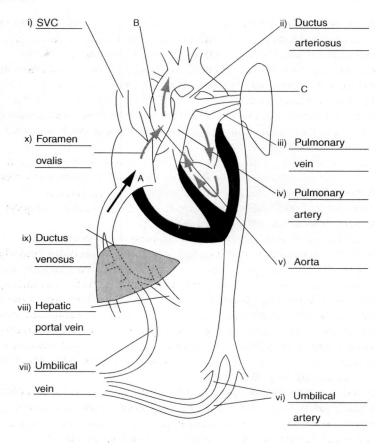

i) SVC

B

ii) Ductus arteriosus

C

x) Foramen ovalis

iii) Pulmonary vein

A

iv) Pulmonary artery

ix) Ductus venosus

v) Aorta

viii) Hepatic portal vein

vii) Umbilical vein

vi) Umbilical artery

(a)   See diagram (the blood goes via the foramen ovale to the left ventricle).
(b)   See diagram.
(c)   There is a higher concentration of oxygen at point B.
(d)   The richer concentration of oxygen supplies the upper body and the fetal head is the part that undergoes most growth in gestation.
(e)   Obliteration of ductus venosus and arteriosus and permanent closure of the foramen ovale.

ANSWER 5

(a) Atrial flutter with 4:1 block.
(b) Ventricular rate of 72 bpm with normal axis. Classical 'saw tooth' waveform with a rate of 288 bpm (ie 4× ventricular rate). Rapid conduction rates 2:1 or 1:1 can obscure the flutter waves, and vagal manoeuvres can slow this down to reveal them.
(c) The QRS complexes are narrow with a normal rate, excluding a ventricular dysrhythmia. There are obvious flutter waves excluding atrial fibrillation. The conduction rate is 4:1 but could be of other ratios (3:1, 2:1 or rarely 1:1).
(d) Possible aetiologies include: electrolyte disturbance (hypokalaemia, hypomagnesaemia); coronary artery disease and ischaemia; systemic hypertension; valvular heart disease; cardiomyopathy, cor pulmonale, and congenital cardiac disease; post-cardiac surgery; thyrotoxicosis; and idiopathic.
(e) Treatment will depend upon whether there is any acute haemodynamic change and of course on correction of the underlying cause. General principles should include supportive measures such as oxygen, fluids and correction of electrolyte disturbances (along ALS guidelines). Rate control is often not a problem in atrial flutter, indeed digoxin can convert atrial flutter into atrial fibrillation, and many drugs that affect AV-nodal conduction are ineffective in this arrhythmia. Therefore, if not self-limiting, cardioversion (usually by synchronised low-energy DCC shock) is often required. Occasionally rapid atrial pacing can be used.
(f) Atrial flutter is often not tolerated well and so rarely becomes chronic without becoming atrial fibrillation. Anticoagulation, therefore, is not normally required per se unless the underlying pathology would otherwise require it (eg post-mitral valve replacement).
(g) The ECG also demonstrates voltage criteria for left ventricular hypertrophy (net V_2 S-wave + net V_5 R-wave height > 35 mm). Note, there is no strain pattern (inverted T-waves in I and aVL).

ANSWER 6

(a) The sacral hiatus.
(b) Skin, subcutaneous fat and the sacrococcygeal membrane.
(c) This is the sacral canal containing the termination of the dural sac at S2 (and filum terminale after this), sacral nerves, coccygeal nerve, internal vertebral venous plexus and fat.

(d)   The two posterior superior iliac spines.

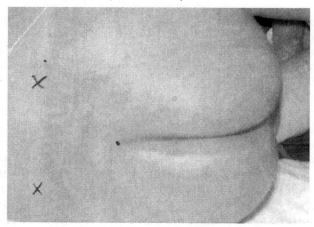

(e)   Likely to terminate at S2.

(f)   May descend to S4.

(g)   16 ml (2 mg/kg).

(h)   1.25 ml/kg. The concentration must be reduced.

(i)   Most commonly the position of the patient is the lateral position with the knees drawn up to the chest. A prone or even seated position could be used. The sacral hiatus is located by feeling for a dimple at the third point of an equilateral triangle formed by the two posterior iliac spines. Using an aseptic technique a needle (or small cannula) is inserted at about 45° to the skin. A click is sometimes felt as the sacrococcygeal membrane is pierced. The needle is directed cranially, the depth being dependent on the size of the patient, although it should not be inserted greater than 2 cm. After inserting the cannula or needle, careful aspiration should be done both initially and after a test dose of 1 ml of local anaesthetic is injected, to confirm the absence of blood or CSF. There should only be minimal resistance to the injection. Increased resistance, subcutaneous swelling and in the awake patient pain can all indicate a periostial or subcutaneous injection.

(j)   Discharge from the ward should only take place after a return of motor function and the absence of urinary retention have been confirmed and once alternative analgesia has been provided.

(k)   It results from a failure of fusion of the 4th and 5th sacral vertebrae.

ANSWER 7

(a) This is a tough station. Your clinical examination needs to be fast and fluent if you are to complete it. The marks will be divided between all the examinations so do not take too long on any individual part. Currently in the exam, you are likely to have a well patient to examine, and the marks are mainly for a thorough technique.

1. Introduce yourself (1 mark)
2. Explain what you are going to do, stress at this stage that if the woman feels at any time uncomfortable or unwell she is to let you know. (1 mark)
3. Positioning of the woman is not essential in this case. However, it is good practice to have a pregnant woman of gestational age greater than 16 weeks reclining and wedged to avoid aortocaval compression. (1 mark)
4. Start with an airway assessment; this should include Mallampati, assessment of movement of head neck and jaw, thyromental and sternomental distance. The presence of large breasts that may require the use of a short-handled blade should be noted. A question to the patient about reflux shows you are aware of the problem. (4 marks)
5. The cardiovascular system should come next. Once again you should follow the same strict system. Inspection should include the hands (looking for splinter haemorrhages, koilonychia, clubbing, etc), eyes (anaemia, arcus, etc), JVP and tongue; also look for sacral and peripheral oedema. The pulse should also be taken at this point. Palpation involves placing your hands over the heart including borders feeling for heaves and thrills. Auscultation should involve listening to all areas of the heart. The patient should be sat forward and the diaphragm and bell of stethoscope used to listen in inspiration and expiration over the aortic area; with the patient in the left lateral position the apex of the heart should be examined with the bell of the stethoscope. Remember to ask to take the blood pressure. (4 marks)
6. Finally the abdominal examination will be performed. Ask the woman to take a breath in before starting the examination and note any scars if you are allowed to expose her. Palpate lightly over all quadrants of the abdomen asking about tenderness; your eyes must be focused on the woman throughout. Calculate the fundal height and try to assess the lie of the baby. A good question at this point is, 'Where do you feel the baby kick?' Ballot the

kidneys and percuss liver and spleen. Auscultate for bowel sounds and listen for renal bruits. You should also state you would like to perform a urine dipstick. (4 marks)

(b) No, this would be high. The normal range is reduced in pregnancy to 25–75 µmol/l.

(c) Yes, see diagram.

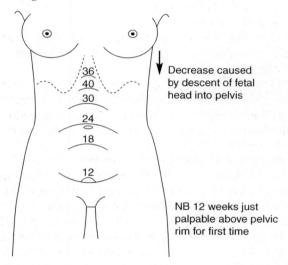

36
40
30
24
18
12

Decrease caused by descent of fetal head into pelvis

NB 12 weeks just palpable above pelvic rim for first time

(d) Yes, this occurs when the baby's head descends into the pelvis.

(e) Yes, this is normal. Pregnant women have an increased minute volume largely due to an increased tidal volume secondary to the central effects of progesterone on the respiratory centre.

(f) Yes, progesterone relaxes the smooth muscle of the vasculature causing a decrease in the SVR.

ANSWER 8

(a) The right subclavian vein is a continuation of the axillary vein and begins at the outer border of the first rib which it then grooves on passing over it. It passes anterior to the subclavian artery separate from it and at a lower level than scalenius anterior (lower owing to the slope of the rib). It runs below the clavicle and subclavius and joins the internal jugular vein at the medial border of scalenus anterior (at the medial end of the clavicle). Important relations include the right lymphatic duct that enters at the angle of confluence of the two veins; the right phrenic nerve which passes between the vein and scalenus anterior; and the pleura of the lung which extends an inch above the medial part of the clavicle, therefore extending both above and below the vein. It is important to note that the vessel is large (at least 1 cm diameter) even in hypovolaemic states, as it is held open by its fixation to surrounding connective tissue.

(b)   As with all practical procedures:

1. You must obtain consent (1 mark)
2. You must ensure access to a trained assistant, appropriate monitoring (in this case at least an ECG) and resuscitation equipment. (1 mark)
3. You must use an aseptic technique. Mention that you would be wearing a hat, gloves, gown, visor and mask. (1 mark)
4. The patient should be positioned head down (to reduce the risk of air embolism) and the head should be turned to the contralateral side. (1 mark)
5. The area needs to be cleaned and draped. (1 mark)
6. The landmark for needle insertion can be found by running a finger from the lateral part of the subclavian groove medially till your finger meets an obstruction, the subclavius muscle, also marked by a notch on the underside of the clavicle. (The subclavius muscle runs from the first rib to the clavicle and provides a reliable landmark for where the subclavian vein lies on the first rib.) This point lies between the midpoint of the clavicle and a point dividing its middle and medial thirds. (3 marks)
7. Local anaesthetic should be placed at the point of insertion. (1 mark)
8. A needle or cannula is then inserted whilst aspirating under the clavicle in the direction of the back of the sternal notch. The needle should be kept close to the underside of the clavicle. Once venous blood has been aspirated, using the Seldinger technique, a wire can be inserted (whilst keeping a close eye on the ECG). The skin and vein are then dilated over the wire and the central venous catheter passed over the top. The line should be sutured in place and a sterile dressing applied. (3 marks)

(c)   Complications include pneumothorax, chylothorax, haemothorax, haemorrhage (this approach is relatively contraindicated in a patient with a coagulopathy as it is not possible to place pressure on the subclavian artery if accidentally punctured and dilated), phrenic nerve injury, air embolism and arrhythmias.

ANSWER 9

(a)

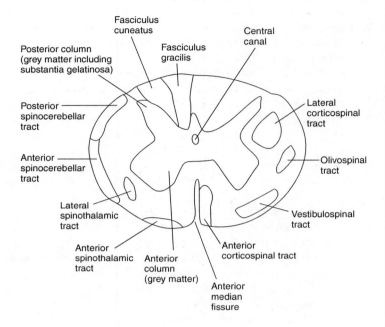

(b) The anterior spinal artery is formed by the union of the vertebral arteries at the foramen magnum and runs down the anterior median fissure and supplies 75% of the spinal cord.
The posterior spinal arteries are formed from the posterior cerebellar arteries and are reinforced by spinal branches of nearby vessels.
The radicular arteries reinforce the supply from anterior and posterior arteries, particularly the *arteria radicularis magna* (artery of Adamkiewicz), which arises distally from the aorta, usually on the left, and is a major supply to the lower two-thirds of the spinal cord.

(c) Destruction of the posterior columns or *fasciculi gracilis* and *cuneatus* causes a loss of fine touch and proprioception (ie joint position sense); the anterior spinocerebellar tracts are responsible for supplying proprioception to the cerebellum.

(d) The lateral spinothalamic tracts decussate close to the point of entry to the spinal cord; in the medulla it joins with the anterior spinothalamic tract to form the spinal lemniscus; this relays in the

164

thalamus before terminating in the cerebral cortex. As a result, somatosensory impulses from one side of the body are represented on the contralateral cerebral cortex.

ANSWER 10

(i)

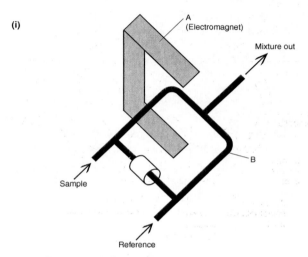

Paramagnetic analyser

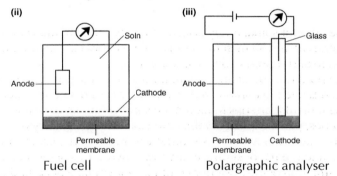

Fuel cell   Polargraphic analyser

(a)   (iii)
(b)   Silver/silver chloride.
(c)   Platinum wire.
(d)   Potassium chloride.
(e)   A gas-permeable, halothane-impermeable plastic covering.

(f)   The electrode requires a voltage to cause an electro-oxidoreduction at the cathode.

(g) $O_2 + 4e^- \rightarrow 2O_2^-$
        $2O_2^- + 2H_2O \rightarrow 4OH^-$

(h) $4Ag \rightarrow 4Ag^+ + 4e^-$
        $4Ag^+ + 4Cl^- \rightarrow 4AgCl.$

(i)   It uses two-point calibration with an oxygen-free reference gas or an electronic zero for the first and 12% O_2 for the second.

(j)   37°C

ANSWER 11

(a)   Facts to establish about the mastectomy:
- Which side is it? (1 mark)
- Has she had any previous surgery, eg axillary clearance, that may restrict cannulation or blood pressure measurement? (2 marks)
- What is the full extent of the surgery, eg does this surgery involve an axillary node clearance? (1 mark)

Establish the nature of the breast cancer:
- Are there any systemic signs suggesting metastases? (1 mark)
- Does she have symptoms of bony metastases that affect her cervical spine? (1 mark)
- Is she receiving chemotherapy, is this having any side-effects, eg nausea and vomiting, pancytopenia, immunosuppression, coagulopathy? (3 marks)
- Does she have any symptoms of anaemia? (1 mark)

(b)   Need to establish exactly what she is prepared to receive, ie all blood products (1 mark), and whether she would be happy to have a predonated autologous transfusion (1 mark). Cell salvage is accepted by some, but is inappropriate here because of the malignancy (1 mark). Does she have any symptoms of pre-op blood loss – ask about haematuria, melaena and haematemesis? (1 mark) Consider deferring surgery for pre-optimisation of haematinics (iron supplementation, erythropoietin). (1 mark)

(c)   Establish from the history the cause of the haematuria (NB these are not necessarily specific to this patient).
1. Clarify that it is from the urethra not the rectum. (1 mark)
2. Congenital, eg haemophilia. (½ mark)
3. Acquired: anticoagulation, risk factors for liver disease, eg alcoholism, hepatitis. (½ mark)
4. Infection: ask about loin pain or dysuria. (½ mark)

5. Tumour: ask about previous employment, eg dye (alanine) workers, or those working with photographic solutions have a higher risk. (½ mark)
6. Stones: history of intense pain in the flank or loin. (½ mark)

Ask about the blood loss.

7. Is there frank blood loss in the urine? (½ mark)
8. How long has it gone on for? (½ mark)
9. What has its effect been on the patient, eg are they suffering from tiredness or syncope? (½ mark)

ANSWER 12

(a) In this situation ventilation should be attempted. (1 mark) The success of the attempt should be maximised by optimising head position and inserting a nasopharyngeal airway. (1 mark)
(b) A cricothyroidotomy should be attempted. (1 mark) A 14G cannula can be used, but many places now have specifically designed emergency airway devices for needle cricothyroidotomy. Most require use of jet ventilation (or at least high-pressure oxygen delivery), eg via a Sanders' injector (ideally with a pressure limiting device). (1 mark) However, some are now wide enough that a conventional circuit can be attached and used to ventilate the patient (Fastrach®).
The cricothyroid membrane can be found by placing the head in a neutral position and palpating the cartilages in the neck in a caudal direction. (1 mark) The first landmark is the notch created by the horns of the thyroid cartilage. A little way below this a less dramatic indentation can be felt; this is the position of the cricothyroid membrane. (1 mark) A syringe with 1–2 ml of saline should be attached to the device, and aspiration applied once through the skin. Two fingers from the other hand on either side of the larynx will help stabilise the trachea and assist placement. The needle or device should be inserted at 90° initially, and then directed more caudally to avoid damaging the posterior tracheal wall (and indeed the oesophagus). (1 mark) Once placement is confirmed through aspiration, the cannula or device can be slid over the needle. Confirmation of endotracheal placement should be done by aspiration on the cannula or device once inserted and if possible by the use of capnography if the device allows. (1 mark) Remember, most expiration with transtracheal jet ventilation occurs via the larynx and oropharynx.
(c) Malignant hyperpyrexia (1 mark)

(d)   1.   **CALL FOR HELP** (1 mark)(The management of malignant hyperpyrexia is incredibly labour-intensive and senior advice should be sought immediately.)

       2.   Emphasise that this is a medical emergency and that a lot of things will be going on simultaneously, which cannot be described in a specific chronological order. (1 mark) Most units have a specific Malignant Hyperpyrexia box or trolley, and it is perfectly acceptable to say that you would require this and to contact the pharmacy for further doses of dantrolene.

       3.   Stop trigger agent if possible, ie shut off vaporisers. (1 mark)

       4.   Surgery should only be continued to achieve haemostasis. (1 mark)

       5.   Switch to a circuit not contaminated with vapour. (Some people question the need for this as vapour will be produced by the patient for a considerable time after the vaporiser has been turned off.) (1 mark)

       6.   Use high flows and hyperventilate the patient with 100% oxygen. (1 mark)

       7.   Remember to keep the patient asleep, usually with an infusion of propofol. (1 mark)

       8.   The key treatment is to give dantrolene 1 mg/kg iv initially. (1 mark) Further increments of 1 mg/kg up to a max of 10 mg/kg can be given; however, if there is no response after 2–3 mg/kg then some recommend reconsidering the diagnosis! Remember dantrolene is relatively insoluble and takes time to dissolve and therefore administer. This is another reason for summoning help at the earliest possible moment.

       9.   Monitor the temperature, and use active cooling methods whilst trying to avoid peripheral vasoconstriction. (1 mark)

     10. Treat the effects of malignant hyperpyrexia: acidosis, hyperkalaemia, coagulopathy. (1 mark)

     11. Instigate invasive monitoring early and watch especially for cardiac arrhythmias and myoglobinuria. (½ mark)

     12. Remember to arrange for an ITU bed. (½ mark)

ANSWER 13

(a)   A brief description of the entire procedure should be given to the assistant.

       ■ A rapid sequence induction is so-named because it involves the rapid administration of an induction agent followed by a muscle relaxant (conventionally suxamethonium) *without* first ensuring the ability to ventilate the patient. (1 mark)

- The intention is to secure the airway in a patient who is not starved or is at risk from aspiration for other reasons (eg small bowel obstruction, hiatus hernia). (1 mark)
- It involves the application of cricoid pressure by the assistant (Sellick's manoeuvre); this works because the cricoid cartilage of the trachea is the only complete ring of cartilage in the larynx, and pressure on this compresses the oesophagus against the cervical vertebrae thereby occluding it without compromising the trachea.(2 marks)

Specific instructions should be given to the assistant.

- The anaesthetic machine should be checked as for any anaesthetic procedure. (1 mark)
- Specific equipment checks include the function of at least two laryngoscopes (either with different size blades or different types of blade); working Magill's forceps; an intact cuff on the endotracheal tube of choice (which should have the inflating syringe preloaded on the pilot balloon) as well as ready availability of a size above and below; a gum elastic bougie should be immediately available to the anaesthetist (often under the patient's pillow); and the suction should be turned on and easily accessible by the anaesthetist. (4 marks)
- The patient needs to be on a tipping trolley and attached to all basic monitoring (ECG, pulse-oximeter, and non-invasive blood pressure) or other more invasive monitoring as the case dictates with good, working intravenous access. (1 mark)

With regards to cricoid pressure, several things need to be discussed: (3 marks)

- The position of the cricoid cartilage can be demonstrated on the patient, the ODP or yourself (often easier than trying to explain it).
- It needs to be applied once consciousness has been lost (eg with loss of eyelash reflex).
- The pressure required is debated. Some advocate the use of 10–20 N awake, followed by 30–40 N once anaesthesia has been induced. How these forces are achieved is beyond the scope of this answer.

Cricoid pressure should not be released until the trachea is intubated, the cuff inflated and adequate ventilation of the lungs ensured (with confirmation by capnography), and a *clear* instruction from the anaesthetist to the assistant to release cricoid pressure is made. (2 marks)

(b) Cricoid pressure can be released when the importance of securing the airway begins to outweigh the risk of aspiration or if the continued application of cricoid pressure may cause potential harm, eg active vomiting can potentially cause oesophageal rupture; misplaced cricoid pressure can cause distortion of the airway and thus compromise the view on direct laryngoscopy. (2 marks)

(c) Once attempts at intubation have been abandoned, the application of cricoid pressure should theoretically be maintained until the patient recovers consciousness. However, the assistant may also be required to help turn the patient in to the left lateral position, or to tip the trolley head down, or both. The ODP may also be required to assist the ventilation of the patient, if this is necessary to avoid hypoxia, whist maintaining cricoid pressure by squeezing the bag or assisting in other ways as directed by the anaesthetist. (3 marks)

ANSWER 14

(a) Nerve injuries can be described by Seddon's classification:
- *Neuropraxia* – this occurs usually as the result of compression or ischaemia of the nerve and is often reversible (2 marks)
- *Axonotmesis* – this occurs often as the result of traction on nerves and relies on there being a preserved Schwann sheath. This is uncommon in anaesthesia and surgery. Recovery may occur depending on the duration of the insult. (2 marks)
- *Neurotmesis* – this is essentially cutting of a nerve. Such damage is often related to the site of surgery and may be intentional, but warning about possible, relevant nerve damage like this should be included in the surgical consent. (2 marks)

(b) General risk factors include obesity, duration of surgery greater than 2 hours, diabetes and prolonged hypotension. (4 marks)

(c) *Ulnar nerve palsy*: leads to a claw hand due to loss of *flexor digitorum profundus* to ring and little fingers; and loss of sensation on the little finger and the lateral (ulnar) border of the ring finger. (3 marks)

Saphenous nerve palsy: leads to loss of sensation to the medial borders of the knee, lower leg and foot. (2 marks)

Common peroneal palsy: leads to foot-drop from impaired ankle dorsiflexion, eversion of the foot and inability to extend the toe; sensory loss to the lateral surface of the leg and the dorsum of the foot. (3 marks)

(d)   Obturator nerve palsy may occur when posts are placed in between the legs in, for example, dynamic hip screw surgery on a traction table. This results in impaired adduction of the thigh and sensory loss on a small area of the medial aspect of the thigh. (2 marks)

ANSWER 15

(a)   The word capnograph comes from the Greek words *kapnos* meaning smoke and *egrava* meaning to write.
(b)   Carbon dioxide is maximally absorbed at the 4.26 μm point in the spectrum of infrared absorption, which is from 1 to 40 μm.
(c)   Nitrous oxide causes a phenomenon known as collision broadening. Energy is transferred from the nitrous oxide molecules, which are vibrating at a higher frequency with more energy than the carbon dioxide. The transferred energy results in an overestimation of the amount of CO_2 present.
(d)

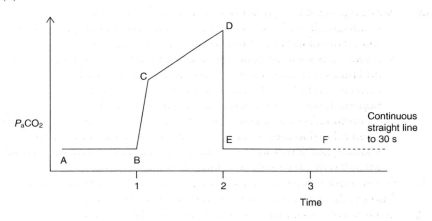

B + C   Dead space and alveolar gas
C + D   Alveolar gas
No: Fowler's method uses the volume of gas plotted against % conc of nitrogen to determine the volume of the anatomical dead space.
(e)   There is no precise point at which you can say inspiration is occurring. The lack of CO_2 measured is *exactly* that – no CO_2 being *measured*. The reasons for this non-measurement of CO_2 include: exhaled dead space gas, the end-expiratory pause and inspiration

itself. Obviously, it also occurs with tube disconnections and obstructions, etc.

(f)   This is true, expiration is occurring at this point.

(g)   This is incorrect as AB includes at least some expiration.

(h)   No CD is up-sloping and this is characteristic of CO_2 release from alveoli with different time constants, for example a patient suffering from chronic obstructive pulmonary disease.

(i)   This is true; see above.

(j)   No, a situation like this affects the initial rise in CO_2 release.

(k)   This is physiologically impossible.

(l)   An air embolism would cause a progressive reduction in CO_2; however, it would not be the abrupt termination shown here.

(m)   Unlikely but possible; a lengthy period like this would suggest a degree of voluntary control therefore raising the possibility of awareness.

(n)   Cerebral hypoxia will occur when all reserves of oxygen are utilised and is certainly not an immediate event.

(o)   True, surgery should be halted if possible until the cause has been ascertained. If the airway has been lost this must be rectified before surgery is allowed to continue.

(p)   This trace is characteristic of an oesophageal intubation.

ANSWER 16

(a)   It would be wrong to assume that the tachycardia is primarily pain related in a hypotensive, pyrexial, barely conscious, acidotic woman.

(b)   The SVR is low; the normal range is 1000–1500 dyne s/cm^5.

(c)   No; if you have diagnosed a patient with septic shock, antibiotics should not be delayed unnecessarily. It would be reasonable to draw off blood for culturing immediately before the administration of the antibiotics.

(d)   The pyrexia, low SVR with high cardiac output and acidosis all support an initial diagnosis of sepsis.

(e)   According to The American College of Chest Physicians (ACCP)/Society of Critical Care Medicine (SCCM) Consensus Conference the definition of sepsis is that of systemic inflammatory response syndrome (SIRS) in the presence of confirmed infection. SIRS has very broadly encompassing, but specific diagnostic criteria. Two or more of the following must be seen in the presence of a known aetiology:

 ■ Heart rate > 90 bpm.
 ■ Core temperature <36 or > 38°C.

- Tachypnoea > 20 breaths per minute or, on blood gas, a $P_aCO_2 < 4.3$ (kPa (32 mmHg)).
- White blood cell count of $<4\times10^9$ or $>12\times10^9$ per litre, or the presence of greater than 10% immature neutrophils.

(f)   The hypotension is very unlikely to be the result of primary myocardial dysfunction (ie left ventricular failure). However, although the cardiac output is high in sepsis, echocardiographically the left ventricle is often somewhat dilated and does not function normally when compared to non-septic patients.

(g)   A fluid challenge would be appropriate. It is the response to filling that is important and in this case the PCWP may be more reliable. Pulmonary oedema is likely over 18–20 mmHg, so a cautious fluid bolus in this scenario would be reasonable.

(h)   This would be an appropriate choice of vasopressor given the low SVR and high cardiac output. The Charing Cross protocol for renal rescue therapy suggests the use of noradrenaline to raise the mean blood pressure and perfuse the kidneys.

(i)   Adrenaline is perhaps not the preferred first-line inotrope, however it is certainly not contraindicated. There is some concern that the use of adrenaline increases lactate levels though the significance of this is uncertain.

(j)   No the pulmonary capillary wedge pressure is high; the normal range is 6–12 mmHg.

(k)   Pulmonary capillary wedge pressure represents the back-pressure from the left atrium, and relies on the pulmonary venous system being normal and unimpeded. It is considered to be a better measure of left ventricular filling pressure that than the use of CVP (which is more representative of right ventricular filling pressures).

(l)   The pulmonary pressures are high (normal systolic 15–30 mmHg and diastolic 0–8 mmHg) and could indicate increased pulmonary vascular resistance; however, this is not explained by the history as given.

(m)   Complications of pulmonary artery (PA) catheters can be divided into the complications of central venous access (for the large PA introducer) and those specific to the PA catheter itself. Complications of central venous access are trauma to other structures in the neck (carotid puncture, tracheal damage, thyroid damage, laryngeal damage, vagus nerve and recurrent laryngeal nerve damage) and local complications such as haematoma formation and infection. If inserted via the subclavian route then subclavian vessel damage can obviously occur, as well as there being a higher incidence of pneumothorax formation. (see question 8). Complications of the PA catheter itself include arrhythmias (both ventricular and supra-ventricular), myocardial perforation (right atrium and ventricle), tricuspid and pulmonary valve damage, pulmonary artery rupture, pulmonary infarction (if balloon is left inflated and wedged), knotting of the catheter (especially in dilated hearts) and infection/endocarditis. Misinterpretation of results can also lead to incorrect therapeutic interventions, which may partially explain the fall from favour of PA catheter usage.

(n)   This is correct. Obviously other clinical and radiological criteria need to be met; however, to diagnose ARDS rather than acute lung injury (ALI), a ratio of arterial concentration of O_2 compared to F_iO_2 needs to be greater than 26 kPa.

(o)   APACHE scoring should not be used for this purpose. It is intended to look at populations and cannot really be applied to individuals to make prognostic decisions.

ANSWER 17

(a)   Mean (4.4) is the average $[(3 + 4 + 6 + 6 + 7 + 2 + 4 + 5 + 1 + 6) \div 10]$. Mode (6) is the value that occurs the most [1, 2, 3, 4, 4, 5, 6, 6, 6, 7]. Median (4.5) is the middle value such that half the data points are below or equal to it and half the data points are greater than or equal to it. [1, 2, 3, 4, 4, 5, 6, 6, 6, 7].

(b)   Subarachnoid classification: nominal
Blood pressure: discrete
Penile length: continuous.

(c)   Positively skewed (hump to right).

(d)   These data show a normal distribution. The key characteristics of this are that the mean, median and mode are numerically the same. Also, 67% of values lie within 1 standard deviation (SD), 95% within 2 SD and 97.5% within 3 SD.

(e)   Student's t-test.

(f)   In a journal containing 20 papers each with a probability value of $P=0.05$, one will have occurred completely by chance.

(g)   A type I or alpha (α) error is said to occur when a difference is proven statistically where one in fact does not exist, ie we incorrectly reject the null hypothesis. ('Now you see it').

(h)   A type II or beta (β) error is opposite to this, ie a statistically significant difference is *not* demonstrated when a difference does in fact exist and we do not reject a null hypothesis when it is in fact *false.* ('Now you don't'). A type-II error is important when calculating the power of a study.

(i) The scatter diagram shows a negative correlation of – 1, ie in this particular example the taller you are the less you would spend on health care.

OSCE 2 – Questions

QUESTION 1

A young couple present to you in the pre-assessment clinic asking about the anaesthetic and possible methods of pain relief their 5-year-old son might receive who is scheduled for a circumcision next week.

(a) Your consultant, whose supervision you will be under, prefers to do an intravenous induction and the parents want to know how you will do this and what the advantages are over an inhalational induction. (10 marks)

(b) Discuss the options for pain relief, describing the pros and cons of each. (10 marks)

QUESTION 2

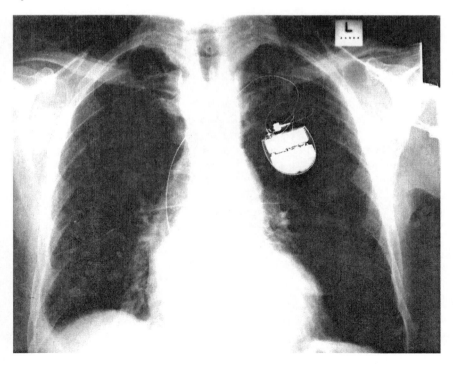

The X-ray above comes from a patient with Marfan's syndrome presenting for a partial gastrectomy for uncontrolled bleeding from a gastric ulcer.

(a)   How is Marfan's syndrome inherited? (1 mark)
(b)   How would you describe the penetration of the X-ray? (2 marks)
(c)   Is the X-ray AP or PA? How can you tell? (2 marks)
(d)   How many posterior ribs can be seen? (1 mark)
(e)   Is the X-ray taken in inspiration? (1 mark)
(f)   Is there evidence of a pneumothorax? (1 mark)
(g)   Is rib notching is present on the X-ray? (1 mark)
(h)   Describe the border of the mediastinum. (2 marks)
(i)   Describe the cardiac border. (2 marks)
(j)   How would the measured blood pressure vary in the arms and legs of the patient? (2 marks)
(k)   Would a regional anaesthetic be the safest choice in this patient? (2 marks)
(l)   If this patient had dental treatment would antibiotic prophylaxis be required? (1 mark)
(m)   Would the patient be more or less likely to be a difficult intubation? Qualify your answer. (2 marks)

QUESTION 3

Sim man question.

Your patient is brought in by ambulance having been found unconscious on a mountain side. His friend, who was out with him, tells you that the patient fell a couple of feet breaking his leg (right tibia and fibula). The friend went to get help and due to poor weather the patient has been out on the mountain side for 12 hours. At the scene the patient had a weak pulse, but now this cannot be felt.

(a)   Describe your initial management. (5 marks)

The rhythm shown on the screen is ventricular fibrillation and the patient's temperature is 28°C.

(b)   How will the patient's physiology be different from normal at this temperature? (10 marks)
(c)   What is important with regards to defibrillation and cardiopulmonary resuscitation? For how long should it be carried out? (5 marks)

QUESTION 4

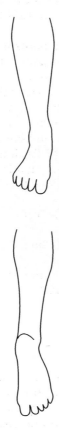

(a) Annotate the diagrams indicating what areas are supplied by which nerves. (NB Actual nerves are required and not dermatomes.) (12 marks)

(b) Describe the course of the saphenous nerve. (3 marks)

(c) What position should the leg be in if you are performing a posterior tibial nerve block? (2 marks)

(d) What is the toxic dose described in the BNF for these local anaesthetics?

    i.   Bupivacaine (1 mark)

    ii.   Plain lignocaine (1 mark)

    iii.   Lignocaine with adrenaline. (1 mark)

QUESTION 5

(a)   Label the parts of the diagram below (3 marks)

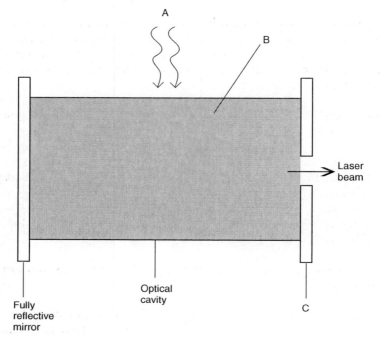

(b)   What does LASER stand for? (1 mark)
(c)   What can provide the energy source? (3 marks)
(d)   What medium produces a laser mainly absorbed by haemoglobin?
       (1 mark)
(e)   What medium is in the Nd:YAG laser and what is it used for?
       (3 marks)
(f)   Which is more combustible N_2O or O_2? (1 mark)
(g)   Why do some goggles say CO_2 only? (2 marks)
(h)   Up to what strength laser are goggles required? (1 mark)
(i)   Does water or haemoglobin absorb most energy at longer
       wavelengths (over 2 μm)? (1 mark)
(j)   Name two changes to the endotracheal tube that can be made to
       improve patient safety. (2 marks)
(k)   What is the bucket of sand used for in a theatre in which lasers are
       used? (1 mark)

QUESTION 6

You are presented with the following scenario:

A 25-year-old man has been involved in a collision with another car coming head on; he was not wearing a seat belt. The ambulance crew needed to call the fire service to remove him from the car, and this has taken over 2 hours. The car was not fitted with airbags and the ambulance crew note a circular crack on the windscreen.

He arrives sitting up and chatting, he says he feels like he has been hit by a truck and he aches all over.

(a)   What should your initial management be and why? (9 marks)
(b)   Demonstrate how you would determine his Glasgow Coma Score (an actor is lying next to the examiner on a couch).

What you would do to perform a painful stimulus? What are the pitfalls of the various approaches? (2 marks)

The actor responds as if one has been applied and grunts, withdraws and opens his eyes to speech.

(c)   Calculate his GCS; what is the significance of this? (5 marks)
(d)   What physical signs may the patient have suggestive of an anterior fossa fracture? (4 marks)

QUESTION 7

You are presented with a 25-year-old man breathing about 40% oxygen via a Hudson mask. He is barely rousable. He has been complaining of low abdominal pain that the surgeon thinks is secondary to an inflamed appendix and has therefore listed him for an appendicectomy. Some biochemistry results are shown:

pH	7.1
PO_2	30.0 kPa
PCO_2	2.5 kPa
BE	−21 mmol/l
HCO_3^-	10 mmol/l
Glu	29 mmol/l

Na+	149 mmol/l
K+	6.0 mmol/l

Urinalysis reveals	glucose +++
	ketones +++
	protein +

(a) This is an example of a partially compensated metabolic acidosis (True/False). (1 mark)

(b) These are classical findings consistent with a deterioration in a patient with type II diabetes (True/False). (1 mark)

(c) Insulin treatment should be the same regardless of whether it is a hyperosmolar non-ketotic (HONK) coma or a diabetic ketoacidosis (DKA) (True/False). (1 mark)

(d) Intravenous morphine 10 mg would be appropriate (True/False). (1 mark)

(e) Rapid infusion of a litre of normal saline would be appropriate (True/False). (1 mark)

(f) The patient will require urgent anticoagulation (True/False). (1 mark)

(g) 250 ml of 8.4% bicarbonate should be given to correct the acidosis (True/False). (1 mark)

(h) He should be given 5% dextrose to correct his hypernatraemia (True/False). (1 mark)

(i) Surgery would definitively treat his abdominal pain and should not be delayed (True/False). (1 mark)

(j) His increased respiratory rate is due to his pain (True/False). (1mark)

(k) Calculate his expected P_aO_2, explaining your reasoning. (3 marks)

(l) List four drugs that could be used to lower a high serum potassium level. (4 marks)

(m) What else should be done if the potassium is over 8.0 mmol/l? (3 marks)

QUESTION 8

(a)   The following cervical spine X-rays are from a patient with rheumatoid arthritis. What features give rise for concern? (4 marks)

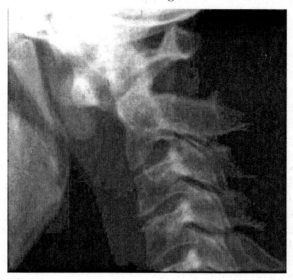

(b)   What features can be seen in this intraoral view? (3 marks)

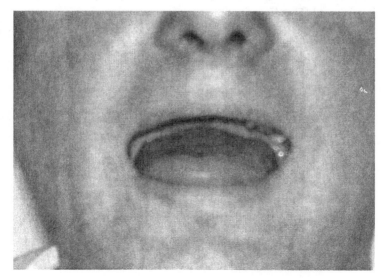

(c)   What components make up Wilson's Score? (5 marks)

(d)   Give five predictors of difficult ventilation. (5 marks)

(e)   The diagram below shows a cross-section of the neck at the level of T2. Indicate the position of the trachea, oesophagus, carotid artery, jugular vein, cephalic veins, sympathetic chain. (3 marks)

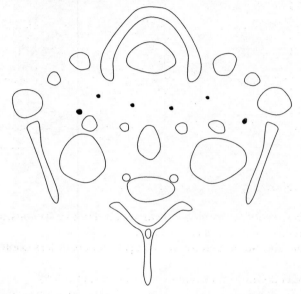

QUESTION 9

A patient is brought into Accident and Emergency. On assessment he has no pulse and a sinus rhythm of 60 bpm on the monitor.

(a)   Describe your immediate management. (4 marks)
(b)   How often should adrenaline be given? (1 mark)
(c)   What should change after the patient is intubated? (1 mark)
(d)   What could be the cause of this situation? (8 marks)
(e)   The rhythm changes to ventricular fibrillation (VF). How would your management change? (4 marks)
(f)   If the patient had arrived in VF and has now been resuscitated to sinus rhythm with a good output, how should you continue his care? (2 marks)

QUESTION 10

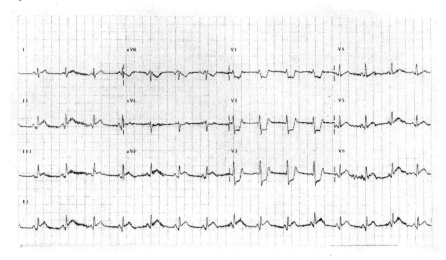

Answer the following True/False questions:

(a) This ECG would most likely be associated with hypotension. (1 mark)
(b) This ECG shows a sinus tachycardia. (1 mark)
(c) The rate should be controlled with β-blockers unless contraindicated. (1 mark)
(d) The ECG demonstrates a normal QRS axis. (1 mark)
(e) This ECG shows features of an acute inferolateral myocardial infarction. (1 mark)
(f) This ECG shows features of an acute posterior infarction. (1 mark)
(g) This ECG shows signs of an acute right ventricular infarction. (1 mark)
(h) This ECG could be in part the result of an occlusion in the circumflex artery. (1 mark)
(i) This pattern on the ECG suggests an almost total occlusion of the left anterior descending artery. (1 mark)
(j) If chest pain suggestive of ischaemia is present, angioplasty should be considered as a first-line treatment. (1 mark)
(k) When considering the effects of a right ventricular infarction, clinical features include clear lung fields, an elevated venous pressure and a positive Kussmaul's sign. (1 mark)
(l) A partial right bundle branch block is present. (1 mark)

(m) The Q-waves in lead II are suggestive of an old myocardial infarction. (1 mark)

(n) The P-R interval is shortened suggesting that the patient has an existing pre-excitable condition. (1 mark)

(o) Any elective surgical procedure should be postponed for at least 6 months. (1 mark)

(p) If operated on within the next 4 weeks the risk of re-infarction is at least 40%. (1 mark)

(q) The commonest time for reinfarction is 3 days postoperatively. (1 mark)

(r) Saddle-shaped S-T elevation throughout leads V_4–V_6 may indicate a pulmonary embolus. (1 mark)

(s) Persistent S-T elevation despite treatment may indicate a ventricular aneurysm. (1 mark)

(t) Papillary muscle damage will initially cause aortic regurgitation. (1 mark)

QUESTION 11

Communication post-anaphylaxis.

A patient (an A-level biology student) anaesthetised by you has had an anaphylactic reaction. (You gave propofol, fentanyl, vecuronium and co-amoxiclav.) Your management in all respects has been perfect and after 3 days on ITU the patient has been extubated. You are informed by one of the nurses on ITU that he is highly distressed and is considering litigation against you for negligence. When you see him he asks you a number of questions.

(a) Is it normal to have nightmares after ITU and what can be done? (3 marks)

(b) What is an anaphylactic reaction? (3 marks)

(c) What caused it? (3 marks)

(d) How do you know it was an allergic reaction? (4 marks)

(e) What could be done to stop it happening to him or anyone else in the future? What tests can be done and how? (7 marks)

QUESTION 12

The following lung function tests are from a lady who is booked in to have a Nissen's fundoplication.

FVC	2.12 l (2.72–3.69)
FEV$_1$	1.68 l (2.18–2.96)
FEV$_1$/FVC	79% (67–80)
PEFR	262 l/min (326–441)
FRC	1.54 l (2.16–2.92)
TLC	3.14 l (3.94–5.33)
VC	2.37 l

(a) Describe briefly what will happen surgically. (3 marks)
(b) What is the definition of FEV$_1$? (1 mark)
(c) What is the definition of FVC? (1 mark)
(d) What pattern do the results suggest? (1 mark)
(e) What makes up the FRC? (1 mark)
(f) How is the FRC measured? Which technique will give the highest value? (4 marks)
(g) Is it important that she is treated with a salbutamol nebuliser pre-surgery? (1 mark)
(h) If the DL$_{CO}$, corrected for both haemoglobin and lung volume, is normal, give three possible causes of the pattern. (3 marks)
(i) What use is the K$_{CO}$ value in this situation? (2 marks)
(j) Below is a normal flow volume loop; superimpose a typical loop for this patient. (3 marks)

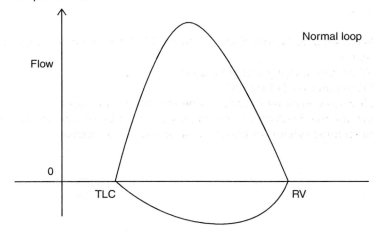

QUESTION 13

You are shown the CT of a man who you have been asked to see in casualty following an alleged assault involving a baseball bat. The scan reveals a *bilateral* fracture of the zygoma and maxilla. He is mumbling incoherently, opening his eyes to pain, and he is flexing his arms in an unusual manner in response to pain. His oxygen saturations are 90%, there is blood in his airway, he appears to be going into laryngospasm and he can no longer be bag mask ventilated despite the use of airway adjuncts.

(a)   Describe a commonly used classification for this type of facial fracture. (4 marks)

(b)   Calculate his Glasgow Coma Score (show the breakdown) (3 marks)

(c)   What bones make up the roof floor and medial and lateral walls of the orbit? (8 marks)

(d)   Should you attempt an awake fibreoptic intubation? (1 mark)

(e)   Is an awake cricothyroidotomy indicated in someone with bilateral zygomatic fractures? (1 mark)

(f)   Is suxamethonium contraindicated? (1 mark)

(g)   Should the oral endotracheal tube be left uncut initially? (1 mark)

(h)   What nerve is likely to be damaged with an injury to the superior margin of the orbit. (1 mark)

QUESTION 14

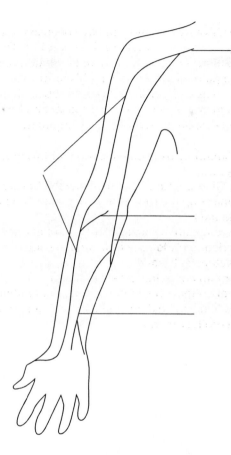

(a)   Label the diagram of the venous drainage of the forearm. (5 marks)
(b)   Which vein is best for the insertion of a long line and why? (2 marks)
(c)   What is the name of the test to assess the collateral ulnar circulation to the hand, what is it used for and how useful is it? (1 mark)
(d)   Describe how you would perform the above test? (1 mark)
(e)   Describe the course of the median nerve. (3 marks)
(f)   What are the relations of the antecubital fossa? (3 marks)
(g)   Where could you block the ulnar nerve in order to anaesthetise only the hand and forearm? What is the disadvantage of blocking the nerve here? (2 marks)
(h)   What precisely is blocked? (3 marks)

QUESTION 15

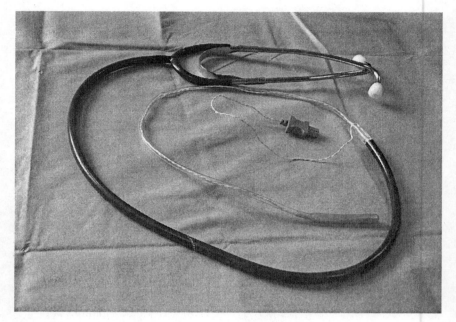

(a) List the information that can be gained from this piece of paediatric monitoring equipment. (5 marks)

(b) What technique of temperature measurement is most commonly used by this equipment? (1 mark)

(c) Draw a graph of temperature versus electrical resistance for the platinum wire electrode. (2 marks)

(d) Name the four processes that lead to heat loss in a patient in theatre. (4 marks)

(e) What is the definition of specific heat capacity? (2 marks)

(f) What are the clinical effects of hypothermia? (6 marks)

QUESTION 16

(a) Take a history from a man presenting for resection of a Duke's B carcinoma of the colon. He is complaining of shortness of breath. He thinks the doctor said he had asthma but he could not be sure. Ask relevant questions to determine the cause. (15 marks)

(b) Explain what the Duke's classification is and its relevance to anaesthesia in terms of prognosis. (5 marks)

QUESTION 17

In a trial, a new drug A is compared against drug B in the prevention of vomiting: 100 people took drug A and 100 people took drug B. The results are tabulated below.

	Drug A	Drug B
Vomiting	40	80
No vomiting	60	20

(a) Could Fischer's exact test be applied to these data? Qualify your answer. (2 marks)
(b) What type of data are they? (1 mark)
(c) What is the absolute risk reduction? (2 marks)
(d) What is the relative risk reduction? (2 marks)
(e) Calculate the odds ratio. (2 marks)
(f) Calculate the numbers needed to treat. (2 marks)

Then, 18 patients from this trial were recruited and this time half took drug A and half took drug B. From each patient 10 temperature measurements were taken at half-hour intervals over the next 5 hours. The researchers expect drug A to reduce temperature in the patients. Answer the following True/False questions:

(g) This is a double-blind trial although it did not involve a placebo. (1 mark)
(h) The data from each group can be assumed to be parametric. (1 mark)
(i) Temperature in degrees centigrade can be regarded as continuous data. (1 mark)

(j)   If confidence intervals contain values from both groups, the null hypothesis can be rejected. (1 mark)

(k)   The confidence interval for group A is based on its standard error of the mean. (1 mark)

(l)   The sample size of the group is inversely related to the power of the test used. (1 mark)

(m)   The Mann Whitney U test would be an appropriate test to compare the data. (1 mark)

(n)   Student's t-test would be inappropriate as it assumes normal distribution of the sample and the population. (1 mark)

(o)   If a Spearman's rank correlation was used the difference would have to be greater to achieve a value of $P = 0.05$. (1 mark)

OSCE 2 – Answers

ANSWER 1

(a) This question does not give you the option of an inhalational technique as a first-line approach. Your answer should follow this rough structure:

Premed – EMLA and Ametop® are both acceptable, but you may be asked the benefits of one versus the other. Explain that although this will not completely remove all sensation it will remove the pain. Suggest that a sedative, eg midazolam, is available if the child is very distressed on the day of surgery, although it may not be appropriate if he is scheduled for day case surgery. (2 marks)

Anaesthetic room – The child will be brought down from the ward with a nurse and usually only one parent, who can stay with him during the first part of the induction period, ie from arrival until enough anaesthetic has been given so that the child is unconscious. (1 mark) The child will be either lying on the trolley or on the parent's lap. The choice for this can be given to the child, giving them some feeling of empowerment. (1 mark) Usually the child will choose the parent's lap. The child will often be positioned so that they are facing the parent with their legs either side and arms wrapped around. This gives an opportunity to cannulate the child out of the child's sight (1 mark). Explain that despite the very best distraction techniques the child may become distressed at this point. You should also say that the attempt at cannulation is limited. If the child becomes very distressed and starts to struggle, you will proceed to a gas induction. This may be done without further discussion and may be distressing to both child and parent. (1 mark) Also say that whatever the method the child will go very floppy as if in a very deep sleep. (1 mark) At this point, they must be transferred without delay to the trolley, if they are not already on it. This is when the parent will be asked to leave. (1 mark)

Advantages – There is evidence to suggest that an intravenous induction is less stressful for the child; it is also arguably safer as the intravenous access provides an immediate and effective route of drug administration. (2 marks)

193

(b)   All postoperative pain relief questions can be answered in this general format. Mention the different types of pain relief:
Simple analgesics: Paracetamol and non-steroidal anti-inflammatory drugs – these are simple analgesics used as an adjunct to all other techniques with very few side-effects. (Don't forget to mention the *per rectum* route). (2 marks)
Weak and strong opiates: These have a tendency to cause nausea and vomiting, constipation and occasionally respiratory depression, any of which may lead to delayed discharge. (2 marks)
Caudal block: You need to mention the risks of a dural puncture headache, increased time to mobilization (heavy legs), increased time to micturition, failure and rare complications such as nerve damage, total spinal with severe hypotension and intravascular injection. (3 marks) However, it is possibly the most reliable technique, which will give good operating conditions. (1 mark)
Penile block: This provides good pain relief; however, it may fail, and there is a risk of nerve damage (numb patch) and intravascular injection. (1 mark)
Topical lignocaine gel: may not be effective; however, it is minimally invasive albeit with the risk of high absorption from a raw area and possibly an increased risk of infection. It is possibly of more use post-discharge. (1 mark)

ANSWER 2

(a)   Marfan's syndrome is a connective tissue disease inherited as an autosomal dominant gene.

(b)   The penetration of the X-ray is perfect as you can just see the lumbar vertebrae outline.

(c)   The chest X-ray is PA; it is of high quality and the scapulae are out of the lung fields.

(d)   6 posterior ribs can be seen.

(e)   The above would only be the case if it was taken in inspiration.

(f)   There is no evidence of a pneumothorax; however, given the history of Marfan's the X-ray should be looked at with this in mind.

(g)   Rib notching is present on the middle parts of the lower border of the ribs posteriorly (this is caused by enlarged collateral vessels).

(h)   The mediastinum shows a double aortic knuckle and a small descending aorta.

(i)   The cardiac border is enlarged consistent with an enlarged left ventricle.

(j)   The blood pressure would be high in the arms and low or normal in the legs.

(k)   Regional anaesthesia would be inappropriate for many reasons: the patient may well have a coagulopathy, be extremely hypovolaemic and the surgery will be intraperitoneal.

(l)   The patient should receive antibiotic prophylaxis as if they had valvular heart disease.

(m)   The patient has an increased risk of being a difficult intubation as Marfan's is associated with a high arched palate.

ANSWER 3

(a)   As always, an ABCDE approach should be taken. (1 mark)
The patient is unconscious and needs to be ventilated, initially with 100% oxygen and as soon as possible the patient should be intubated. (1 mark)
Chest compressions should be commenced and the patient linked to a cardiac monitor. (1 mark)
At this point the patient's temperature should be taken. (1 mark)
Intravenous access should be secured and slow rewarming commenced as soon as is practicable. (1 mark)

(b)   Hypothermia affects our physiology in a different in a number of ways:
Cardiovascular – The patient will be severely vasoconstricted, and at 28°C is likely to be in refractory ventricular fibrillation (ie not amenable to shocking). The cardiac output (if not in arrest) will be reduced by 30% at 30°C. (3 marks)
Respiratory – There is a left shift of the oxygen dissociation curve, a reduced O_2 requirement and decreased CO_2 production. (2 marks)
Central nervous system – Below 30°C the patient will be unconscious with a reduced cerebral metabolic rate. It is partly for this reason that the saying, 'a patient is not dead until warm and dead' exists, as hypothermia gives cerebral protection and may improve outcomes. (2 marks)
Other – There is usually a degree of coagulopathy, a reduced glomerular filtration rate, increased blood viscosity and haematocrit, hyperglycaemia and metabolic acidosis. (3 marks)

(c)   Warming and continuous cardiopulmonary resuscitation are as important as defibrillation at very low temperatures because the rhythm is likely to be refractory to shocking or drug therapy. (1 mark)
Warming should be quick until a temperature is reached such that a sustainable cardiac rhythm has been achieved, and thereafter at 1°C per hour. (1 mark)

Techniques of rewarming should include warmed fluids (nasogastrically, intravenously, intraperitoneally or via the urinary catheter), and external warming devices (eg warm air devices, warming mattresses, although direct warming is not advised as it may burn vasoconstricted skin). Warming of inspired gases with the use of an HME and possibly other humidification systems may also be of benefit. In extreme situations, if available or feasible, use of cardiopulmonary bypass may be possible. (3 marks)

ANSWER 4

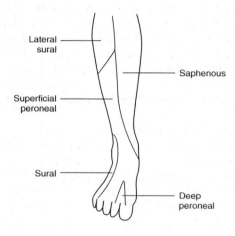

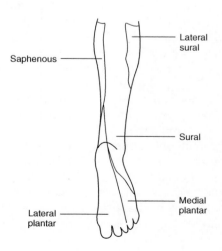

(a)   The *tibial nerve* divides into medial and lateral plantar nerves behind
       the medial malleolus supplying the medial and anterior parts of the
       sole of the foot. The *sural nerve* runs behind the lateral malleolus and
       supplies the posterior part of the sole, the back of the lower leg, the
       heel and lateral aspect of the sole of the foot. The *deep peroneal
       nerve* supplies the area between the 1st and 2nd toes. The *superficial
       peroneal nerve* supplies the dorsum of the foot. The *saphenous nerve*
       supplies the medial aspect of the medial malleolus. The cutaneous
       branch of the *common peroneal nerve* supplies a V-shaped wedge of
       skin above the lateral malleolus.

(b)   The saphenous nerve branches off from the femoral nerve in the
       femoral triangle below the inguinal ligament. It runs initially laterally
       to the femoral artery before moving medially. It then descends
       between gracilis and sartorius. Finally it passes down the medial
       border of the tibia in front of the medial malleolus.

(c)   The patient should be supine with the leg externally rotated. It can
       also be blocked higher up in the popliteal fossa, when the patient
       should be prone.

(d)   The correct maximum doses are:

     i. Bupivacaine   2 mg/kg
     ii. Plain lignocaine   3 mg/kg
     iii. Lignocaine with adrenaline   7 mg/kg.

ANSWER 5

(a)   A. Energy source; B. Laser medium; C. Partially transmitting mirror.

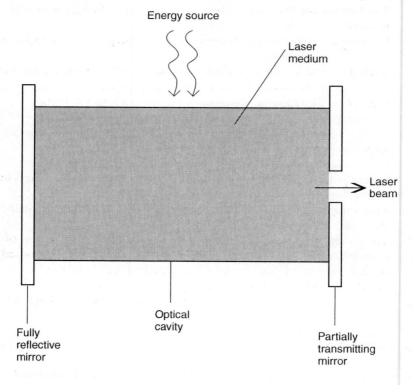

(b)   Light Amplification by the Stimulated Emission of Radiation.

(c)   An electric discharge of high voltage, a flash of intense light from a flash tube or another laser.

(d)   The blue green argon laser is mainly absorbed by substances coloured red. It therefore avoids damaging transparent structures and is useful in coagulating vessels in the retina for example.

(e)   Nd:YAG stands for neodymium:yttrium-aluminium garnet. It is a solid medium that produces a near-infrared laser which is absorbed deeply into the tissues; it is ideal for debulking tumours.

(f)   Nitrous oxide is far more combustible.

(g)   Protective goggles must be appropriate to the wavelength of the laser in use. CO_2 in particular has a wavelength of 10,600 nm, more than a hundred times longer than most lasers, making these goggles even more specific.

(h) Up to Class IIIa.

The international classification of continuously working lasers is as follows:

Class I –   Powers do not exceed the maximum permissible exposure for the eye.

Class II –   Refers to a visible beam powered up to 1 mW; for this the eye is protected by the blink reflex time.

Class IIIa – This category is a relaxation of class II to 5 mW for radiation provided that the beam is expanded and protected by the blink reflex.

Class IIIb – for powers up to 0.5 W. Direct viewing of this is hazardous and protective eye wear is required.

Class IV – for powers over 0.5 W which are extremely hazardous to the eye.

(i) Water has a higher relative absorbance at wavelengths greater than 2 µm.

(j) There are a number of options: cuffs filled with dye or saline; use of double-cuffed tubes; aluminium or copper tape around the standard tube; and metal or specific laser tubes. Metal tubes have the disadvantage that there is no cuff.

(k) This is used as a receptacle for a burning plastic tube resulting from an airway fire.

ANSWER 6

(a) A trauma call should be put out. He may be chatting but there is a high index of suspicion that the patient has sustained a significant injury. The circular crack on the windscreen is known as a 'bullseye' and is associated with significant head and neck injury. The history of a 2-hour extraction is also associated with significant forces involved in the incident and therefore significant injury. (3 marks)

ABCDE approach should be taken followed by a secondary survey.

Airway and C-spine control – Given the history the patient's spine must be immobilised.

Breathing – Hi-flow oxygen via Hudson mask with reservoir, saturation monitoring and a chest X-ray should be performed.

Circulation – At least two large-bore cannulae (avoiding limbs with obvious injury), blood pressure and ECG monitoring.

Disability/pain – His pain should be treated and his initial Glasgow Coma Score (GCS) assessed; in this case it is initially 15.

Environment – The ambient temperature should be raised if he is exposed for any length of time and he should be covered when at all possible. When assessment is complete warm air devices can be used. (5 marks)

Following this a secondary survey should be performed which will consist of a head to toe examination front and back, including a rectal examination. (1 mark)

(b) A painful stimulus needs to be modified depending on the situation. Pressure to the nail bed alone is unlikely to be satisfactory as the patient may not respond due to a spinal injury. A sternal rub may not be appropriate in the face of a significant chest injury. Generally, painful stimuli should be central and not in the area of any injury.

(c) Eye opening to speech scores 3 points; withdrawing to pain scores 4 points; incomprehensible sounds scores 2 points.

Total GCS is 9/15.

This is a large drop from the initial GCS on arrival, suggesting a significant head injury, and is an indication for an urgent CT. Most people would advocate intubating the patient at this point, as although the GCS itself would not mandate airway protection, it has fallen rapidly and is likely to do so further. In addition it would be appropriate to control his CO_2 in the face of likely intracranial damage.

(d) Nasal bleeding, CSF rhinorrhea, peri-orbital haematoma, and any injury of cranial nerves I–IV all indicate a possible anterior fossa fracture.

ANSWER 7

(a) *True* This is an example of a partially compensated metabolic acidosis.

(b) *False* This is a picture of diabetic ketoacidosis in a patient with type I diabetes. The patient has a high serum glucose, ketones in the urine and a profound metabolic acidosis.

(c) *False* In extremis type II diabetics are usually more sensitive to insulin than type I diabetics. A bolus of insulin is not required for the treatment of a HONK and the amount of insulin in a sliding scale is at least 50% less than the amount required for a patient in DKA.

(d) *False* This would be inappropriate in a patient who was barely rousable.

(e)   *True* A litre of 0.9% saline would be a good initial choice of fluid.
(f)   *False* It is the HONK patients who require anticoagulation due to their persisting hyperosmolar state.
(g)   *False* This is an enormous volume of sodium bicarbonate. The evidence for giving sodium bicarbonate in this situation is highly controversial. Though the arterial pH may improve, an *intracellular* acidosis may develop.
(h)   *False* 5% dextrose is rarely indicated. Using such a hypotonic fluid in this scenario risks the development of central pontine myelinolysis.
(i)   *False* Surgery may not cure the pain as the abdominal pain may have originated as a result of the diabetic ketoacidosis. The patient must be resuscitated before surgery is even considered.
(j)   *False* His increased respiratory rate is likely to be in an attempt to compensate for the metabolic acidosis.
(k)   This is about the alveolar gas equation:

$$P_aO_2 \quad = \quad P_iO_2 - P_ACO_2/RQ \qquad \text{(simplified)} \qquad (1)$$

$$P_iO_2 \quad = \quad (101 \text{ kPa} \times 0.4) - 6.3 \text{ kPa} \qquad (2)$$

$$= \quad 34.1 \text{ kPa}$$

$$P_aO_2 \quad = \quad 34.1 \text{ kPa} - 2.5/0.8 \text{ kPa} \qquad (3)$$

$$= \quad 34.1 - 3.125$$

Therefore,

$$P_aO_2 \quad = \quad 34.1 - 3.125 \qquad (4)$$

$$= \quad \textbf{30.975 kPa.}$$

His actual P_aO_2 (30 kPa) is almost identical to the expected value showing that he has no obvious problems in oxygenation.
(l)   Sodium bicarbonate, salbutamol, insulin and glucose can all be used to move potassium into the cell. Calcium resonium can be used in the overall excretion of potassium. Intravenous calcium chloride or gluconate are often used in cardiac arrest due to high potassium levels, but they do not lower the serum level, they simply act as a membrane stabiliser.

(m) At this level the potassium is dangerously high, so calcium chloride or gluconate should be given as myocardial protection (see above), the patient should be monitored on a cardiac monitor, moved to ITU and placed on either haemodialysis or haemodiafiltration.

ANSWER 8

(a) The following is a radiologists report on the X-ray shown. Whilst no one will expect you to provide this level of detail *per se*, it gives a good guide as to roughly what the examiners will be looking for. The changes seen in rheumatoid disease are probably fair game!

There is no patient information on the film. (1 mark)

Lateral view is only from C1 to C4/5 disc space. The C7/T1 junction not visualised (i.e. it is an adequate view). (1 mark)

There is widening of the distance between the anterior arch of the atlas and the odontoid process of the axis, in keeping with anterior atlantoaxial subluxation. The vertebral alignment is otherwise normal. (Think about the potential anaesthetic/airway implications.) (1 mark). There is also widening of the inter spinous distance at C1 and C2 suggesting posterior longitudinal ligamentous instability.

There is minor loss of the anterior disc space at C3/C4 with end plate sclerosis and marginal osteophytes. Some resorption of the tips of the spinous processes is noted. (The latter is possibly artifactual.) (½ mark)

These are features compatible with rheumatoid arthritis. (½ mark)

(b) A clear intraoral view should reveal the uvula, tonsillar pillars and soft palate, as well as the tongue and back of the oropharynx (ie Mallampati I). This view is Mallampati III: only the tongue and soft palate can be seen.

(c) Wilson's Score gives a score of 0–2 for each of the following: weight, head and neck movement, jaw movement, receding mandible and presence of buck teeth. A score of 3 or more predicts around 75% of difficult intubations.

(d) The five predictors of difficult bag mask ventilation are summarised by the acronym OBESE: Obese, Bearded, Elderly, Snoring and Edentulous.

(e)

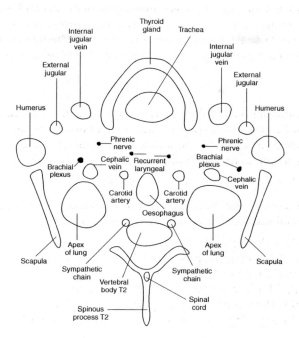

ANSWER 9

(a) Put out a cardiac arrest call. (1 mark)
Start ventilation with 100% oxygen and chest compressions in a ratio of 30:2. (2 marks)
Obtain iv access and give 1 mg adrenaline. (1 mark)

(b) Adrenaline should be given every 3–5 min.

(c) Compressions should become continuous.

(d) 4 Hs & 4Ts:
Hypoxia, hypovolaemia, hypothermia, hypo/hyperkalaemia
Toxins, thrombosis (coronary or pulmonary), cardiac tamponade, tension pneumothorax.

(e) Check pulse, administer a shock of 150–200 J (biphasic), 360 J (monophasic), consider antiarrhythmics (amiodarone) and continue adrenaline and compressions as before.

(f) According to the European Resuscitation Council 2005 Guidelines, patient with out-of-hospital VF arrests should be cooled to 32–34°C for 12–24 hours, and transferred fully monitored to intensive care.

ANSWER 10

(a) *True* This ECG shows a posterior infarction complicated by an inferolateral infarction. This widespread picture of damage could well be associated with hypotension.

(b) *False* This is defined as a rate greater than 100 bpm this is only 90 bpm.

(c) *True* Unless contraindicated, eg pre-existing respiratory disease or severe hypotension, β-blockers would be beneficial to myocardial perfusion by decreasing the oxygen requirements of the heart and increasing perfusion by increasing diastolic time.

(d) *True* The QRS axis is normal.

(e) *True* There is ST elevation present in the inferior leads II, III and aVF. ST elevation also exists in the lateral leads V_5 and V_6.

(f) *True* The posterior infarct is seen as a mirror image of the injury in the septal leads V_1–V_3.

(g) *False* There are no features in this ECG. It can be diagnosed by ST elevation of > 1 mm in lead V_4R (placed in the *right* 5th intercostal space mid-clavicular line).

(h) *True* Although more commonly supplied by the right coronary artery, a dominant left circumflex may supply the posterior descending artery.

(i) *False* An occlusion of the left anterior descending artery will lead to features of an acute anterior infarction, eg widespread ST elevation in leads V_1–V_6.

(j) *True* Primary angioplasty has been shown to be more effective than thrombolysis; however, this is only the case where it can be provided without significant delay (> 1 h after the onset of pain).

(k) *True* These are the features of a right ventricular infarction, with the addition of hypotension.

(l) *False* No bundle branch block is present.

(m) *False* The Q waves in II are less than 2 mm deep and 1 mm across. They are therefore not significant.

(n) *False* The P-R interval is within normal limits (120–220 ms).

(o) *True* This is consistent with current guidelines.

(p) *True* The risk of reinfarction is 40%–60% within this timeframe. Such an event is associated with a very high mortality.

(q) *True* The 3rd night is associated with the return of REM sleep and a sympathetic outpouring increasing the demand made on the myocardium.

(r) *False* Saddle-shaped S-T elevation is more commonly associated with pericarditis 4–6 weeks after an infarct. This can be part of Dressler's syndrome (pericarditis, pleurisy and pneumonitis).

(s)   *True* Persistent S-T elevation may indicate a ventricular aneurysm.
(t)   *False* Papillary muscle damage is associated with mitral valve regurgitation.

ANSWER 11

The actor in this scenario will be acting as an angry difficult patient. DO NOT fall into the trap of becoming defensive. It might not be your fault! You may think it irrational for the patient to be blaming you, but by becoming confrontational, as in real life, this approach will stop the flow of information and your ability to help the patient come to terms with what has happened. So, translating this to the exam you will waste time not communicating the information that will score you marks. The other thing to note is that the question mentions that he is an A-level biology student allowing some room for use of technical terms. However, this is a *communication* station and therefore you must make sure that the terms you use are understood.

(a)   Explain that although not normal, it is not rare. Nightmares often represent a form of post traumatic stress disorder and this could be due to the initial event or his time on ITU. State that you will arrange an appointment with the ITU consultant or follow-up service, if available, to discuss things further. It would be useful to mention that counselling and psychiatric help with or without medication may be required.
(b)   Explain that anaphylaxis is a life-threatening condition. It is usually caused by repeated exposure to an antigen (a particle that is recognised as foreign by the body) which causes the body's immune system to produce antibodies. These are also known as immunoglobulins, in this case a specific type called IgE. [Remember, an *anaphylactoid* reaction requires no prior exposure and is not antibody mediated.] These immunoglobulins bind together on the surface of mast cells causing them to release their contents. The histamine and other substances (kinins, 5-HT and leukotrienes) are then released into the bloodstream. These cause the clinical effects of bronchospasm (tight chest), hypotension (low blood pressure) and oedema (fluid in the tissues).
(c)   The cause of anaphylaxis is difficult to determine from the history alone. However, the likely candidates are co-amoxiclav or vecuronium. The other drugs are very unlikely (although allergy to the egg phosphatide in the emulsification agent is possible). Latex allergy cannot be ruled out and it would be worth taking a history with respect to this.

(d)   The initial diagnosis is made on clinical signs (bronchospasm, urticaria, oedema, cardiovascular collapse). Diagnosis is confirmed with blood histamine and mast cell tryptase levels taken at 1, 6 and 24 hours post-event (NB It is very important that the samples are taken to the lab on ice) and methylhistamine in the urine.

(e)   Explain there is no way to guarantee this will not happen to him or anyone else, as it is a rare and largely unpredictable event. However, you have sent a yellow adverse reporting card so that if this is happening frequently the problem can be identified.

In order for him to know what it was he reacted to and thus avoid future exposure to the allergen, he needs to have the allergen identified. Options for this include:

i. *Radioallergosorbent testing (RAST)* This is only useful for suxamethonium and latex. It involves the use of specific antibodies to antibodies produced as a result of exposure in the serum of the patient.

ii. *Intradermal or skin prick allergen testing* This can be done after 4 weeks and should be done in a centre that has resuscitation equipment available. Dilute samples > 1 in 100 are used with a saline control. A positive test is repeated with a 1-in-10 dilution for confirmation. Steroids do not affect the test. If an allergen is identified this should be documented clearly in the notes and the patient should have a 'medic-alert' bracelet. If the allergen turns out to be commonly encountered then consider giving the patient a preloaded adrenaline syringe (eg EpiPen®).

ANSWER 12

(a)   The top of the stomach is wrapped around the base of the oesophagus where it is used as a noose to restrict the movement of fluid from stomach to oesophagus by acting as a one-way valve. The procedure can be performed laparoscopically and open.

(b) FEV_1 (forced expiratory volume in 1 second) is the maximal volume exhaled in 1 second starting from a maximal inspiration.

(c)   FVC (forced vital capacity) is the maximal volume exhaled after a maximal inspiration.

(d) $FEV_1/FVC = 80\%$. This is a normal ratio yet both FEV_1 and FVC are reduced; this is therefore a restrictive pattern.

(e)   FRC is the functional residual capacity. All capacities are made up of two or more volumes, in this case the residual volume and the expiratory reserve volume.

(f)   FRC can be determined by helium dilution, nitrogen washout and total body plethysmography. The highest value will be achieved from the body plethysmograph as it includes areas that may have little or no gas exchange.

(g)   A salbutamol nebuliser is unlikely to be beneficial in someone with purely restrictive lung disease.

(h)   This will occur where the cause of the restriction is extra-pulmonary: it could be due to pleural effusions, obesity, neuromuscular disorders or spinal or thoracic abnormalities.

(i) K_{CO} helps differentiate conditions in which there is a reduction in surface area which is normal (eg pneumonectomy) from those where the surface area may be reduced, but there is abnormal alveolar membrane (eg emphysema).

(j)

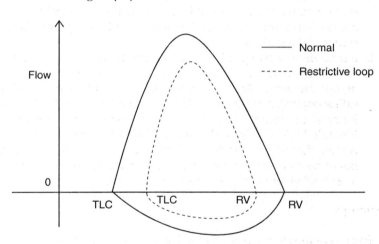

ANSWER 13

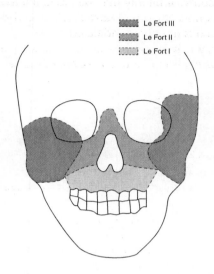

Le Fort III
Le Fort II
Le Fort I

(a) The most commonly used classification is the Le Fort classification of facial fractures. Rene le Fort described a pattern of facial fractures at the turn of the last century which he arrived at by striking the skulls of cadavers with a wooden club or dropping them from a considerable height. The classification is divided into three: Le Fort I, which separates the palate from the maxilla; Le Fort II, which separates the maxilla from the face, and Le Fort III, which results in craniofacial dysjunction.

(b) Eyes open to pain scores 2
Verbal response scores 2
Motor response scores 3
Total score is 7/15.

(c) The margins of the orbit are: medial margin – inferiorly the posterior lacrimal crest of the lacrimal bone and superiorly the frontal bone; lateral margin – frontal process of the zygomatic bone; superior margin – frontal bone; inferior margin – medially the anterior lacrimal crest of the maxilla, laterally the frontal process of the zygomatic bone.

(d) Fibreoptic intubation (awake or asleep) is unlikely to be of use in this sort of situation because of the likelihood of there being unpredictable anatomy and poor conditions because of blood, etc.

(e)   An awake cricothyroidotomy may be indicated in facial trauma;
        however, it is unlikely to be required for isolated zygomatic fractures.
(f)   Suxamethonium is not contraindicated.
(g)   As with burns, where there is likely to be excessive facial swelling the
        tube should be left uncut until the extent of the swelling can be
        determined.
(h)   The supraorbital nerve.

ANSWER 14

(a)   See the diagram below.

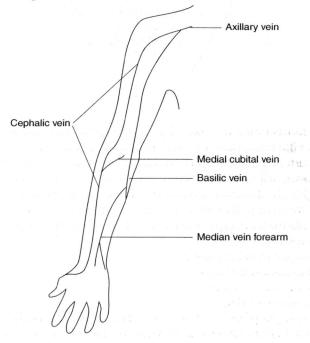

(b)   The basilic vein is the best as it continues to become the axillary
        vein. The cephalic vein joins the axillary vein at an angle and this
        may cause problems in feeding the catheter.
(c)   Allen's test is used to assess whether there is an adequate blood
        supply to the hand from the ulnar artery and therefore whether it is
        safe to potentially occlude the radial artery with a cannula. It is
        extremely unreliable!

(d)   The hand is elevated in a clenched position and the radial artery and ulnar arteries occluded. At this point the ulnar artery is released and the hand is observed to see whether it reperfuses. It should be repeated releasing the radial artery too.

(e)   The median nerve arises from the medial and lateral cords of the brachial plexus (C6–T1). Initially it runs anterior to the axillary artery, then laterally, and finally it crosses the brachial artery at the mid-humerus level to become medial in the antecubital fossa. It continues on top of the *coracobrachialis* and *brachialis* passing under the bicipital aponeurosis and enters the forearm between *flexor digitorum profundus* and *superficialis* lying eventually lateral in the wrist running under the flexor retinaculum and terminating in medial and lateral branches.

(f)   The superior border is formed from a line joining the two epicondyles; the inferomedial border is formed by *pronator teres*, the inferolateral by the *brachioradialis*; the roof is made by fascia (bicipital aponeurosis) and the floor is formed by *supinator* laterally and *brachialis* medially.

(g)   The ulnar nerve can be blocked as it passes behind the medial epicondyle. However, there is a risk of nerve damage both because of direct injury and secondary to nerve compression as there is very little room for the volume of local anaesthetic in this location. There are also some concerns about direct neurotoxicity of the local anaesthetic as the nerve is relatively unprotected by fat and subcutaneous tissue.

(h)   From the elbow distally, the nerve provides motor supply to flexor *carpi ulnaris*, *flexor digitorum profundus* (medial part), the intrinsic hand muscles (except two lateral lumbricals and thenar muscles); it also supplies sensation to the little and medial half of the ring fingers, and the medial part of the hand both on the dorsal and palmar aspect.

ANSWER 15

(a)   Heart rate, respiratory rate, quality of heart sounds (intensity, rhythm, murmurs) and diagnosis of respiratory disorders (pulmonary oedema, bronchospasm, presence of secretions, ventilator disconnection).

(b)   Theoretically any one of the three electronic (platinum wire, thermocouple and thermistor) methods could be used; however, the thermistor is least cumbersome and therefore most commonly used.

(c)   The platinum wire resistance increases linearly with an increase in temperature.

(d)   The four processes are conduction, convection, radiation and evaporation.
(e)   The specific heat capacity of a substance is the energy required to raise the temperature of a substance 1 kg in mass by 1°C.
(f)   Mild clinical effects:
- Shivering (increases metabolic rate and oxygen consumption, which can lead to increased stress and the risk of cardiac ischaemia).
- Problems with wound healing and an increased rate of wound infections.
- Decreased metabolism of drugs (decreased hepatic blood flow).
- Any hypothermia will lead to a left shift of the oxygen dissociation curve and a decrease in oxygen delivery to the tissues compounding the above problems.

More severe clinical effects:
- Decreased level of consciousness.
- Coagulation disorders.
- Metabolic acidosis.
- Life-threatening arrhythmias.

ANSWER 16

(a)   There are a number of things to cover in this question:

- Ask the patient about his symptoms of breathlessness, ie duration, progression, exacerbating/relieving factors, associated symptoms, eg chest pain, exercise tolerance. (5 marks)
- Ask about presence of cough, whether there is anything produced, and specifically colour of sputum (1 mark) or presence of blood (1 mark).
- Specific asthma-related questions should include medication, whether or not he gets relief from his salbutamol (blue) inhaler (the answer no may indicate a respiratory disorder without a reversible component) (1 mark); hospital admissions, particularly those requiring ventilation (1 mark); how well it is controlled (1 mark); and triggering/relieving factors. (1 mark)
- Smoking history should always be asked. (1 mark)
- Allergies. (1 mark)
- Occupation, eg mining, work with asbestos. (1 mark)
- Pets, eg keeping birds. (1 mark)

(b)   Duke's A – tumour confined to the rectal wall, no spread beyond
      muscularis mucosa.
      Duke's B – the growth has breached the rectal wall.
      Duke's C – the regional lymph nodes are involved.
      Duke's D – distant spread has occurred, eg to the liver. (3 marks)

It has obvious relevance to anaesthesia as the prognosis from a
Duke's B that turns into a Duke's C is at least three times lower. So
any postponement must be kept to a minimum and weighed up as to
whether it will achieve a significant benefit for the patient. (2 marks)

ANSWER 17

(a)   No, although it is a version of the Chi-squared test (which would be
      appropriate here) Fischer's exact test is primarily used for small
      numbers (typically less than 20).
(b)   Nominal.
(c)   80%–40% = 0.4.
(d)   (80%–40%)/80%= 0.5.
(e)   (40%/60%) / (80%/20%) = 0.17.
(f)   1/absolute risk reduction = 1/0.4 = 2.5.
(g)   *True* The stem implies that both drugs are unknown to both patient
      and researchers and would therefore be a double-blind trial. Whether
      the trial contains a placebo is irrelevant to whether it qualifies as a
      double-blind trial.
(h)   *False* The data from such a small sample are unlikely to be
      parametric. The data should at least be plotted out before they can be
      assessed.
(i)   *True* Temperature in degrees centigrade could be considered
      continuous.
(j)   *True* This would lead to a rejection of the supposition that both
      groups are from different populations.
(k)   *True* This is a reasonable assumption.
(l)   *False* The sample size is directly related to power.
(m)   *True* Mann Whitney *U* test is the correct choice to analyse two non-
      paired groups of continuous non-parametric data.
(n)   *True* It is inappropriate for those reasons.
(o)   *True* Spearman's Rank is for unpaired ratio data, therefore *P* values
      are higher.

OSCE 3 – Questions

QUESTION 1

(a) Look at the following pictures and state what problems there are with the set up of this arterial line. Explain the effects these errors will have on the readings. (20 marks)

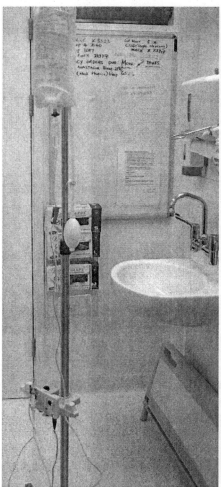

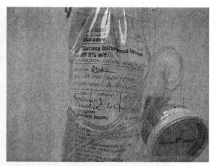

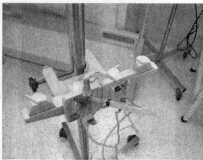

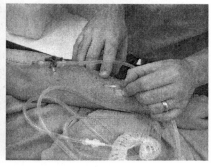

QUESTION 2

Examine the respiratory system of this patient.

Explain to the examiner which parts of the respiratory system the different parts of your examination are testing. (20 marks)

QUESTION 3

You are asked to assess an obese man for an appendicetomy. He tells you that recently he has been suffering from chest pain.

(a)   What relevant factors in the history and examination in relation to his obesity do you need to plan your anaesthetic? (12 marks)
(b)   Obtain a more detailed history about his chest pain. (4 marks)
(c)   What is your differential diagnosis for the chest pain? (4 marks)

QUESTION 4

Sim man

You are called by a nurse on the ward as she has just witnessed a patient collapse onto the bed.

(a)   Describe your initial management. (4 marks)

The patient's blood pressure is 80/40 mmHg with a pulse rate of 40. He is unresponsive to pain.

(b)   What is your differential diagnosis of the bradycardia? (6 marks)
(c)   How should you now tailor your management *pharmacologically*? (3 marks)
(d)   If it was suspected that the patient had taken a β-blocker overdose what is your treatment? (1 mark)

There is no response to your initial pharmacological management and now the patient is showing signs of heart failure.
(e)   What is your next line of management? (2 marks)
(f)   What are the indications for a permanent pacemaker? (3 marks)

QUESTION 5

A patient arrives in A & E with a number of empty bottles which his wife has collected from his bedside. She tells you that two of the bottles were full that morning: diazepam, which he takes to calm his nerves, and imipramine, which he has for his depression and to sleep at night.

He has a fluctuating level of consciousness; his Glasgow Coma Score (GCS) is 12/15 (Eye opening: 3; Verbal response: 4; Motor response: 5). The patient says to you in a lucid period that he wants to be left alone and if you continue touching him he will call the police and have you arrested for assault.

Answer the following True/False questions (1 mark each)

(a) Treatment of this patient constitutes assault.
(b) Flumazenil should be given to improve his GCS.
(c) Expected clinical signs include miosis, urinary retention and dry skin.
(d) Activated charcoal should be given immediately.
(e) The patient requires immediate intubation.
(f) Imipramine's toxic effect is due to:
  ■ an antidopaminergic effect
  ■ an indirect adrenergic block
  ■ a membrane-stabilising effect on the myocardium
  ■ a serotonergic effect
  ■ an anticholinergic effect.
(g) The ingested dose of imipramine and diazepam is a good indicator of prognosis.
(h) An ECG should be done eventually but should wait as initially it is not helpful.
(i) Arrhythmias that develop should be treated with procainamide or quinidine.
(j) Heart block may occur as a result of toxicity.
(k) Alkalinisation should be used to treat CNS complications.
(l) The blood should be alkalinised to a pH of at least 7.4.
(m) Hypertonic saline has been used successfully to treat associated cardiac problems.
(n) Hartmann's solution would be a reasonable choice of fluid to correct hypotension.
(o) Problems with hyperkalaemia often occur in this situation.
(p) If no symptoms have occurred within 6 h and the psychiatrist is happy to discharge, then the patient can go home.

QUESTION 6

This station is based on the photograph shown, of a man with an enlarged anterior pituitary as a result of an expanding tumour.

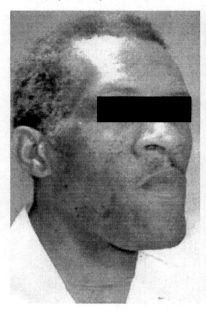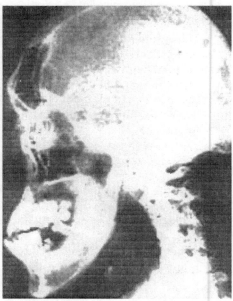

He has recently complained of increasing shortness of breath, an inspiratory wheeze and a change in his voice. On examination, he is noted to have a postural drop in his blood pressure. Answer the following questions. (1 mark each)

(a) What condition is this man suffering from?
(b) Does he have hypoadrenalism, otherwise known as Conn's syndrome?
(c) Would his ability to move his lower incisors past his top incisors make him a class A?
(d) Is he likely to have a high or low Mallampati score?
(e) On examination his soft palate can be partially seen making him grade IV (True/False).
(f) His longer than average thyromental distance is likely to be predictive of a difficult airway (True/False).
(g) His longer than average sternomental distance is likely to be predictive of a difficult airway (True/False).

(h)   The patient has noticed a change in his voice over the last year and now has some difficulty in breathing, and has stridor. Would you consider fibreoptic intubation to be the best method to secure the airway? Would this decision negate the need for further investigation?

(i)   These patients are often hypoglycaemic (True/False).

(j)   The patient is taking bromocriptine; could this be the cause of his postural hypotension?

(k)   The X-ray shows evidence of trauma to his frontal bone (True/False).

(l)   There is a clear pneumocephalus on the X-ray (True/False).

(m)   Would you consider a CT of his neck to be an essential preoperative investigation?

(n)   Cushing's syndrome is clearly present in the photograph (True/False).

(o)   Comment on the sella turcica.

(p)   He may be suffering from tunnel vision (True/False).

(q)   Is he likely to suffer from diabetes insipidus secondary to an increase of ADH production?

(r)   What is affected more by an excess of growth hormone, bone or soft tissues?

(s)   Is he likely to snore?

(t)   Is he at greater risk of pressure area damage?

QUESTION 7

You are asked to see a very anxious biology student in the very early stages of labour. She has heard about epidurals as a means of pain relief but knows very little about them. She wants to know everything about the anatomy and the insertion.

(a)   Discuss the pain relief options, other than epidural, which are available in labour and the advantages and disadvantages of each. (7 marks)

(b)   Describe what you would do to insert an epidural needle into the epidural space and the anatomical layers the needle actually goes through. (6 marks)

(c)   Explain the complications associated with an epidural and give an indication of the likelihood of these complications occurring. (7 marks)

QUESTION 8

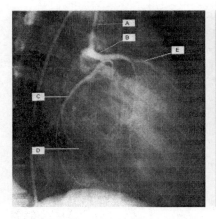 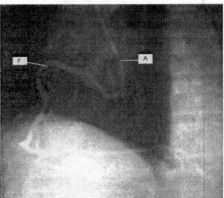

Study the above angiogram and answer the following questions.

(a)   What is A? (1 mark)
(b)   What is B? (1 mark)
(c)   What parts of the myocardium does B supply? (3 marks)
(d)   What is C? (1 mark)
(e)   What is D? (1 mark)
(f)   What is E? (1 mark)
(g)   What is F? (1 mark)
(h)   Triple vessel disease refers to which vessels? (1 mark)
(i)   Which vessel usually supplies the sino-atrial node? (2 marks)
(j)   Which vessel supplies the atrio-ventricular node? (2marks)
(k)   What is the sensory supply to the pericardium? (1 mark)
(l)   What is the autonomic supply to the myocardium? (2 marks)
(m)   Describe the course of the parasympathetic nerve supply from the brain to the myocardium. (3 marks)

QUESTION 9

Study the following pictures concerning the readings from the monitor shown below.

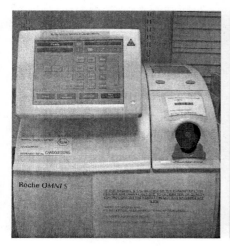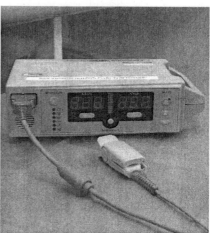

(a) What does monitor A measure? (1 mark)
(b) What can it be used to assess? (3 marks)
(c) How does a co-oximeter differ from a clinical pulse oximeter? (3 marks)
(d) How is the arterial blood flowing in the finger assessed by A? (2 marks)
(e) What potential sources of error exist in using this device? (6 marks)
(f) What is happening to the trace below? (1 mark)

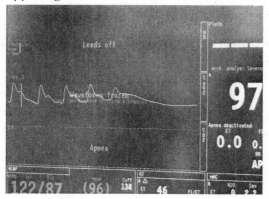

(g)   What else carries oxygen? (1 mark)
(h)   What is the significance of the following points on the graph? (3 marks)

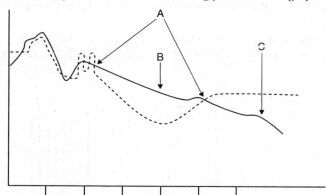

QUESTION 10

(a)   Fill in the details on the table below (12 marks)

Group	Incidence (%)	Red cell antigen	Plasma antibodies
A			
B			
AB			
O			

(b)   What sort of antibody is involved in an ABO incompatibility reaction? (1 mark)
(c)   Could O-positive blood be given to a B-negative woman in an emergency if there was no O-negative available? What are the potential consequences? (3 marks)
(d)   What is in SAGM? What role does it play in storage? (4 marks)

QUESTION 11

The following question involves the use of diathermy in theatre

(a)   What type of current is used in diathermy? (1 mark)
(b)   What alternatives are there to diathermy? (4 marks)

(c) Why is the patient not always electrocuted by the use of diathermy?
     (3 marks)
(d) What needs to be considered when a diathermy plate is used?
     (3 marks)
(e) Why does muscle contract when diathermy is used? (1 mark)
(f) What mode of diathermy is being used in A and B and C? (2 marks)

A

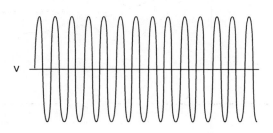

B

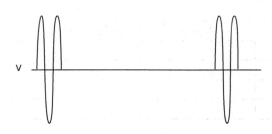

C

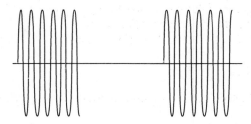

(g) Discuss the undesirable effects that can result from the use of
     diathermy. (6 marks)

QUESTION 12

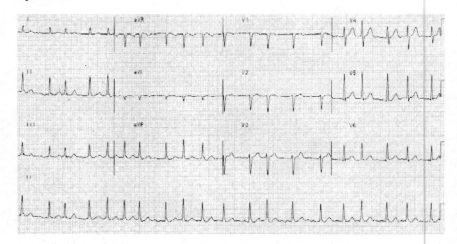

You are asked to assess an 80-year-old woman in the resuscitation room with a history of severe COPD and ischaemic heart disease. She has a blood pressure of 150/80 mmHg, pulse 150 beats/min and her ECG is shown above.

(a)   What is the rhythm on the ECG? (1 mark)
(b)   What are the causes of this condition? (4 marks)
(c)   What classes of drug therapy are available to control the rate? (5 marks)
(d)   Which specific drugs would be contraindicated and why for this lady? (4 marks)
(e)   How much is the cardiac output reduced in this state? (1 mark)

On review, prior to giving rate-controlling drugs, you note that her BP is 80/40 mmHg, she is experiencing chest pain and has basal crepitations. You proceed to cardioversion.

(f)   What is important about the mode of shock and what does this avoid? (3 marks)
(g)   What energies should be used for a monophasic defibrillator? (1 mark)
(h)   What energies should be used for a biphasic defibrillator? (1 mark)

QUESTION 13

Look at this picture of the base of the skull.

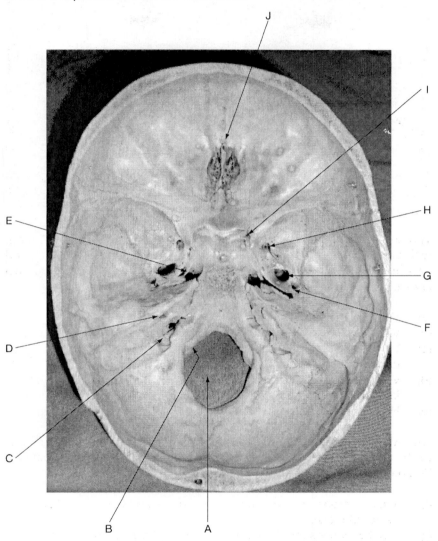

(a) What are the foramina and structures shown and what passes through them? (20 marks)

QUESTION 14

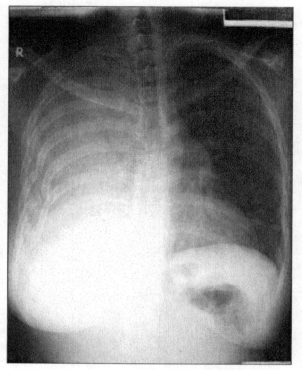

(a) Is this X-ray adequately penetrated? (1 mark)
(b) What gender is the patient? (1 mark)
(c) What radiological abnormalities are shown? (2 marks)
(d) What do these radiological findings indicate clinically? (1 mark)
(e) What important steps should be taken in the management of this condition? (4 marks)
(f) Which mode of analgesia would be most effective in the treatment of pain in this condition? (1 mark)

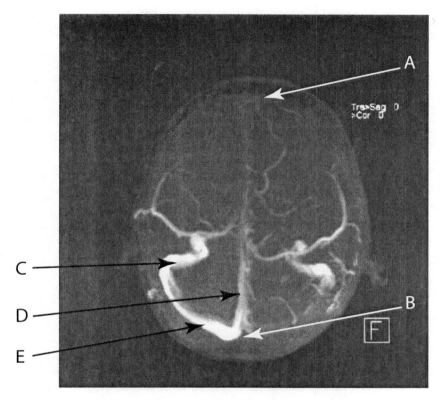

(g) What radiological investigation has been performed? (1 mark)
(h) What abnormality is shown? (1 mark)
(i) What membrane lies between A and B? (1 mark)
(j) What structures are denoted by the letters C, D and E? (3 marks)
(k) What structures meet at D? (1 mark)
(l) Describe the circulation of cerebrospinal fluid within the brain. (3 marks)

QUESTION 15

This ECG is taken from a man with chest pain.

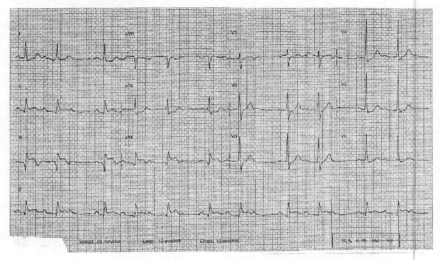

(a) Report this ECG. (5 marks)
(b) Give three common causes of the conduction abnormality. (3 marks)
(c) Is there evidence on the ECG that the patient should be given antibiotic prophylaxis to protect against endocarditis? (1 mark)
(d) Is there any evidence that the patient has deranged potassium on the ECG? (1 mark)

This ECG is taken from a 28-year-old man with Down syndrome.

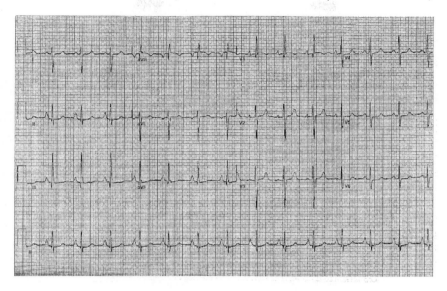

(e)   Describe the ECG (4 marks)
(f)   What cardiac abnormalities are commonly associated with Down syndrome? (5 marks)
(g)   The man presented with cyanosis. What syndrome could he have developed? (1 mark)

QUESTION 16

The following tracings were recorded from women in labour. Read the clinical descriptions and then go on to answer the questions.

Trace A

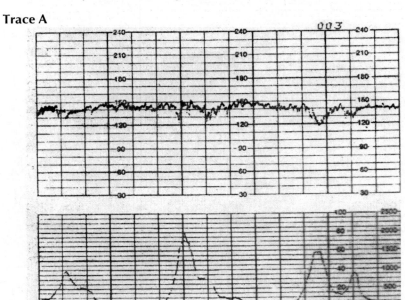

Trace B

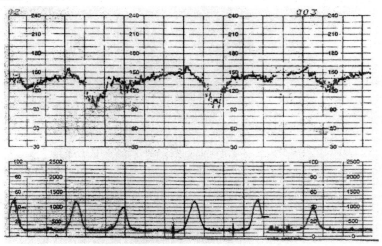

Trace C

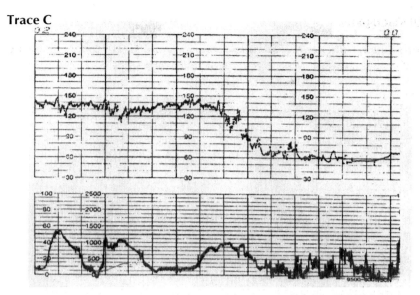

Trace A is taken from a woman well into her second stage of labour.

(a) What does CTG stand for? (1 mark)
(b) What is the normal fetal heart rate range? (2 marks)
(c) What does the bottom trace measure and what are the units?
     (2 marks)
(d) The woman has been booked for theatre. Does the CTG trace
     concern you? What would you do if you were concerned? (3 marks)

Trace B is also taken from a woman in the second stage of labour.

(e) Does it give any cause for concern? (3 marks)

Trace C occurs after an epidural top-up is given in the delivery room by a
very junior midwife. Answer the following questions:

(f) You should inform the obstetrician (True/False). (1 mark)
(g) The trace is unlikely to recover, therefore the woman should be
     transferred immediately to theatre (True/False). (1 mark)
(h) The epidural dose could have gone intrathecally (True/False). (1 mark)
(i) The woman should be placed in the right lateral position (True/False).
     (1 mark)

(j)   Fluid alone may correct the trace (True/False). (1 mark)

(k)   If a drug is required to support the blood pressure ephedrine would be preferred to phenylephrine (True/False). (1 mark)

(l)   If the trace continues to look like this, the woman should be topped up and undergo a caesarean section (True/False). (1 mark)

(m)   The trace is an example of a temporary perfusion phenomenon commonly seen with epidural usage (True/False). (1 mark)

(n)   The baby is born with a heart rate of 50 bpm, apnoeic, blue, flaccid and demonstrates no reflexes; this corresponds to an Apgar score of 2 (True/False). (1 mark)

QUESTION 17

A new cancer drug A is to be compared to cancer drug B in a trial. The week the trial starts, a paper is published showing a significant improvement in outcome with drug A, reducing mortality by 50%.

(a)   The trial can only continue after all of the patients that have been recruited are informed (True/False). (1 mark)

(b)   The trial should continue and the results analysed at intervals; if the same results are produced, the trial should be terminated (True/False). (1 mark)

(c)   The trial should be abandoned (True/False). (1 mark)

(d)   A historical control could be used (True/False). (1 mark)

(e)   The trial is 'one-tailed' (True/False). (1 mark)

The funding for the trial is withdrawn. However, a drug company steps in with the means to finance a new trial comparing drug C (a brand new drug) against drug A.

(f)   Describe the phases required to bring drug C into clinical practice. (12 marks)

Data are also collected on the average blood concentration of the drug and time taken to discharge from hospital.

(g)   Outliers that distort the correlation should be removed when analysing the data (True/False). (1 mark)

(h)   If data turn out to be skewed it is reasonable to modify them mathematically (True/False). (1 mark)

(i)   A correlation value of 0.9 proves that a high concentration of drug leads to a long hospital stay (True/False). (1 mark)

OSCE 3 – Answers

ANSWER 1

(a)   The faults are as follows:

- *No pressure in bag*. This will allow blood to backtrack up the line, which will eventually clot, rendering the set useless. (2 marks)
- *Fluid used is 5% dextrose with 40 mmol potassium chloride*. The use of 5% dextrose, because it is hypotonic, may cause localised haemolysis; the use of potassium may cause localised vasospasm; both increase the risk of ischaemia. Some people argue that you do not even need to use heparinised saline for arterial flush systems. (3 marks)
- *The cannula is too large*. The unnecessarily large cannula may be difficult to insert and will obstruct the flow of blood distal to the cannula. It would also affect the harmonics of the system. (2 marks)
- *Intravenous giving set*. This has the potential to lead to drug errors with the administration of intravenous drugs intra-arterially. (2 marks)
- *Bubbles in line*. This would increase damping giving a falsely low systolic and high diastolic reading. (2 marks)
- *Very long tubing*. This increases the natural frequency of the system giving a reading which will oscillate excessively round a true reading (falsely high systolic and falsely low diastolic). (2 marks)
- *The cannula is in fact intravenous*. This should be obvious! The cannula is not in the brachial artery and therefore will not give a reading. (2 marks)
- *The three-way tap has been left open, connecting patient to air*. This can lead to haemorrhage, which may be concealed beneath drapes, etc. (2 marks)
- *The transducer is too low*. This will give an artificially high reading. It can be calculated by converting the height in cmH_2O to mmHg. (2 marks)
- *Insertion by a practitioner not wearing gloves*. This increases the risk of infection and the transmission of communicable diseases. (1 mark).

ANSWER 2

Here you are likely to have a healthy actor as a patient. The emphasis is on a slick but thorough examination, structured technique and appropriate reporting of negative findings. It may be worth asking the examiner whether he or she would like you to give your findings as you go or save them to the end. Establish whether you are allowed to ask the patient any questions. Remember this is an examination station NOT a history taking one; in this question there are no marks for the history and this must be the assumption unless you are told otherwise. Finally try to decrease the number of times a patient is asked to sit back and forward, for example if you have just finished percussing the patient's back, start your auscultation of the back.

Follow the routine of inspection/observation, palpation, percussion and auscultation. Remember to expose the patient's chest. The patient in the exam will almost certainly be a man!

Observation

- Introduce yourself and expose the patient to the waist. (1 mark)
- *General* – look for cachexia, shape of the chest and spine, scars, use of expiratory muscles, signs of distress (2 marks) and respiratory rate (1 mark).
- *Hands* – clubbing, tobacco staining, character of the pulse (bounding CO_2 retention), flap or tremor of hypercarbia, koilonychia. (2 marks)
- *Head and neck* – tongue for cyanosis, nicotine staining of teeth, height of JVP and signs of right heart failure, anaemia, ask the patient to speak to assess hoarseness. (2 marks)

Palpation

- Assess adequacy of chest expansion. Expansion should be equal on both sides; a decrease in expansion indicates pathology on that side. Assess front, top, back and base. (3 marks)
- Extend the patient's neck to palpate the trachea in the suprasternal notch. A deviation will denote most commonly a fibrosis or collapse on the side of the deviation. Rarely, it will be pushed over by a large effusion, tumour or tension pneumothorax (the last is unlikely to occur in the exam!) (1 mark)
- Examine the neck for cervical lymphadenopathy. (1 mark)
- For completeness, you should test for tactile fremitus by placing the sides of the hands on the chest and asking the patient to say '99'

repeatedly as you move your hands over the chest wall front and back. This is increased by consolidation and decreased by fluid or air. (1 mark)

Percussion

- Remember to compare sides, front and back. You should percuss the clavicle directly. (2 marks)
- A dull tone suggests consolidation, pleural thickening or fibrosis. A stony dull tone is classically found with a pleural effusion. A resonant tone usually suggests air, ie a pneumothorax or bulla.

Auscultation

- Listen over all areas of the chest front and back with the diaphragm of the stethoscope, except over the apex of the lung (above the clavicle) where the bell is commonly used. (2 marks)
- You may want to mention added sounds; for example, wheeze (inspiratory and expiratory), crackles or rales, and stridor (inspiratory) (you should not need a stethoscope to identify stridor!); diminished sounds, which tend to occur when there is an obstruction to sound, eg obesity, or an obstruction to flow, eg occluded or collapsed airways; or any other sounds, for example pleural rubs or bronchial breathing.
- Vocal fremitus (similar to tactile fremitus but performed by listening over the chest whilst the patient says '99') and whispering pectoriloquy (which entails asking the patient to whisper not phonate whilst listening) are perhaps somewhat outdated. However, it is probably wise to at least mention that you would like to perform them. Where there is consolidation the sound will be more easily heard. (1 mark)
- Finally you should mention that ideally you would want to see a chest X-ray, perform a peak expiratory flow measurement and look for a sputum sample! (1 mark)

ANSWER 3

(a)   Obesity is a multi-system disease. Divide you answer into an
      organised structure.
      ■ *Assessment of obesity* Weight, height and calculate body mass
        index, BMI = weight (kg)/height^2 (m). (1 mark)
      ■ *Airway* Obesity, particularly morbid obesity, is associated with
        difficulty in both ventilation and intubation. Previous anaesthetic
        history may reveal problems, and the patient themselves may have
        been told of previous airway difficulty. In addition, obesity is
        associated with hiatus hernia and questions relating to this should
        be asked. (2 marks)
      ■ *Snoring* Many obese patients will suffer from obstructive sleep
        apnoea (OSA) syndrome. If the patient has a partner, it is likely
        that he has been told precisely the pattern of his snoring. Evidence
        of apnoeic periods or day time somnolence would give rise to
        concern and would ideally be further investigated if time allows.
        Postoperative invasive monitoring and respiratory support such as
        continuous positive airway pressure (CPAP) or non-invasive
        ventilation (NIV) should be considered. (2 marks)
      ■ *Respiratory system* The obese patient is prone to hypoxia due to
        increased O_2 demand, increased CO_2 production, a reduced
        functional residual capacity (FRC) and increased closing capacity.
        Exercise tolerance is a good measure of global respiratory function,
        and breathlessness at rest should ring warning bells. (2 marks)
      ■ *Cardiovascular system* A long history of sleep apnoea symptoms
        may lead to pulmonary hypertension. Ask about ankle swelling,
        episodes of dizziness or breathlessness. They are also more prone
        to systemic hypertension, diabetes, hyperlipidaemia and
        hypercholesterolaemia and thus are at increased risk of peripheral
        vascular and coronary artery disease. (3 marks)
      ■ Other questions should be related to symptoms of diabetes, gout,
        arthritis, hepatic impairment and a history of previous DVT.
        (2 marks)

(b)   If a patient mentions chest pain in *any* context the following
      questions should be asked – site, character, radiation, severity, onset,
      duration, relieving/aggravating factors, associated symptoms
      (palpitations, breathlessness, blackouts, etc). (1/2 mark each)

(c)   The list for the differential diagnosis is long. However, it should
      include ischaemic pain, musculoskeletal pain, pericarditis,
      oesophageal pain (eg oesophageal spasm), pulmonary embolism,

pneumothorax, infection (eg pneumonia), aortic dissection or upper abdominal pain, eg pancreatitis or reflux oesophagitis. (1/2 mark each)

ANSWER 4

(a) Your initial management should be to shake the patient to elicit a response. If this is unsuccessful, call for help. An ABC approach must be taken (1 mark). Open the airway, check breathing, and give high-flow oxygen. Check a pulse and establish some monitoring, especially an ECG (3 marks).

(b) The differential for a bradycardia is heart block, a junctional arrhythmia or a sinus bradycardia caused by a normal physiology (eg sleep), vagal stimulation (eg visceral stretching), hypoxaemia, drugs (eg β-blockers), blockade of cardiac sympathetic innervation (eg high epidural) or disease (eg myocardial infarction).

(c) The patient has a bradycardia and is hypotensive. The European Resuscitation Council (ERC) guidelines should be followed in this scenario. Intravenous access should be secured, if not already, and 500 µg of atropine should be given; vital signs should be reassessed and if there is still bradycardia and hypotension, further boluses of 500 µg of atropine up to 3 mg should be given. Other drugs should be considered including adrenaline, salbutamol, isoprenaline and other β1 agonists, aminophylline.

(d) In this scenario glucagon should be given.

(e) The next line of management would probably involve pacing. This may initially be transcutaneously, via pads, but bear in mind this is only tolerated if the patient is at best semi-conscious. Temporary transvenous pacing should ideally be arranged at the earliest opportunity.

(f) Indications for a permanent pacemaker include symptomatic heart block (eg bifascicular, trifascicular, or complete heart block), any atrioventricular block with sick sinus syndrome, alternating left bundle branch block (LBBB) and right bundle branch block (RBBB), and with implantable defibrillators or overdrive pacing of tachyarrhythmias where there is carotid sinus hypersensitivity.

ANSWER 5

(a)   *False* This is not assault as the patient has not demonstrated that he has informed consent. Also, it could be argued that even if he were to give consent, then, in view of the fact that he has allegedly taken an overdose, he is not mentally capable of giving consent, and therefore any treatment is done in the patient's best interests.

(b)   *False* Guidelines issued by Toxbase® (part of the Health Protection Agency and run by the National Poisons Information Service) state that flumazenil should not be given in a mixed overdose. In addition, giving flumazenil to a patient who has been on long-term benzodiazepines is a potentially harmful act as it is likely to provoke a seizure.

(c)   *False* The anticholinergic effects of a tricyclic antidepressant (TCA) overdose will cause dry skin and urinary retention; they will also cause a mydriasis.

(d)   *False* The evidence for a beneficial effect of activated charcoal given within an hour of the overdose is not conclusive. In this scenario we have no idea when the overdose was taken. It is also a high-risk strategy in a patient with a fluctuating GCS to give them a large volume of charcoal without first protecting their airway.

(e)   *False* On clinical grounds and from an airway point of view alone, there is no immediate concern for the protection of his airway. However, it may be necessary should he require activated charcoal (see above) or if a stomach washout is advised by the local poisons unit.

(f)   The toxic effect of a TCA overdose *is* multifactorial. It is due to their anticholinergic effect, the blocking of re-uptake at adrenergic receptors, a quinidine-like effect that blocks sodium channels leading to a membrane-stabilising effect, and a direct adrenergic block.
- *False*
- *False*
- *True*
- *False*
- *True*

(g)   *False* Ingested doses of drugs are a poor guide to prognosis as the history is often misleading and there is a wide range of the degrees of physiological effects exhibited by patients taking the same dose of a drug.

(h)   *False* The QRS interval is a good predictor of severity. A QRS length >0.16 s denotes a severe overdose.

(i) *False* Quinidine and procainamide are both sodium-blocking drugs and will worsen arrhythmias. All drugs from 1a and 1c should be avoided.

(j) *True* Heart block may occur along with a wide variety of ventricular arrhythmias.

(k) *False* Alkalinisation of the blood will not treat CNS complications, only cardiac ones.

(l) *True* This would be a reasonable target. At this pH, excretion and protein binding of the drug are promoted.

(m) *True* This helps reverse the sodium-blocking action of tricyclic antidepressants.

(n) *True* This is a reasonable choice as the small amount of potassium in it will help correct any existing hypokalaemia.

(o) *False* The reverse is true as the condition is associated with hypokalaemia.

(p) *True* In terms of the pharmacological effects of the overdose, if there are no symptoms after 6 h, the patient could go home. Obviously, the psychological effects need to be considered.

ANSWER 6

(a) The condition is most likely the result of a growth-hormone-producing tumour of the anterior pituitary gland leading to acromegaly.

(b) No. Hypoadrenalism is known as Addison's disease.

(c) Yes, it would.

(d) There is no indication that he would necessarily have either. However, the history and condition suggest that soft tissue changes in the oropharynx may have occurred, and that he may have a large tongue obscuring your view and hence a higher score.

(e) *False* If the soft palate can be partially seen this would make him a grade III.

(f) *False* Less than 6.5 cm is difficult, and his is likely to be longer.

(g) *False* Less than 12.5 cm is difficult.

(h) Fibreoptic intubation is not the solution for all difficult airway problems! The history is more suggestive of a vocal cord problem or subglottic stenosis. In fact, attempts at fibreoptic intubation in these conditions may cause complete occlusion. The airway should be imaged further with a CT scan of his neck.

(i) *False* Hyperglycaemia is more likely as the secretion of growth hormone causes insulin resistance.

(j)   *True* Bromocriptine can cause postural hypotension.

(k)   *False* His frontal bone shows frontal bossing as a result of his acromegaly. There is no sign of trauma.

(l)   *False* This is an enlarged frontal air sinus.

(m) Yes. See answer to 'h' above.

(n)   *False*

(o)   The pituitary sits in the sella turcica or 'Turkish saddle' and this is likely to be enlarged as a result of the tumour.

(p)   True. This occurs with pressure on the inside of the optic chiasma.

(q)   No. Diabetes insipidus results from a *lack* of ADH.

(r)   It affects soft tissues almost exclusively, obviously depending on the age of onset.

(s)   Yes! Increased soft tissue in the oropharynx is likely to cause snoring and possibly sleep apnoea.

(t)   Yes he is.

ANSWER 7

(a)   Other options for pain relief during labour include:
- Entonox
- Transcutaneous electrical nerve stimulation (TENS)
- Acupuncture
- Homeopathy
- Hypnotherapy
- Opiates/patient-controlled analgesia (PCA)
- Local block, eg pudendal nerve blockade
- Spinal anaesthesia
- Water births

The advantages and disadvantages of the above techniques are open somewhat to interpretation. However, as far as measured pain relief is concerned, only entonox and local techniques, including spinals and epidurals (and indeed combined techniques), have been repeatedly demonstrated to have *efficacy* in labour pain relief. The other techniques, including things like breathing techniques, may help labouring women *cope* with the pain, but have limited, if any, analgesic effect. Most techniques obviously have the advantage that they are relatively non-interventional. Opiates have little effect on the pain of labour, but tend to sedate the mother and therefore make the pain more bearable; this of course can be perceived as a beneficial effect even though there is no true pain relief.

In an exam situation, don't be too controversial; explain the different techniques, but stress that some should possibly be more appropriately referred to as coping strategies! (7 marks)

(b) Epidural insertion

- Note: the question only asks about the *needle* insertion!
- The answer to this should follow the structure for any regional technique: informed consent, intravenous access, resuscitation equipment available, patient positioning, anatomy, landmarks and special points. The first part of this (informed consent, etc) needs to be said, even though it is probably taken for granted. Patient positioning (lateral or seated) is usually a matter of individual choice; however, you should state your own preference. (1 mark)
- The level of a lumbar epidural for labour is a choice of L2–L3, L3–L4, or L4–L5. Ideally, especially if a combined technique is used, the lower the epidural is sited the better, as it reduces the risk of spinal cord trauma. A line from the top of the iliac crests (the supracristal or Tuffier's line) usually marks the body of L4. (1 mark)
- The needle should be inserted under sterile conditions by using suitable cleaning solution for the skin, sterile drapes and the anaesthetist wearing a mask and hat, sterile gown and gloves. (1 mark)
- The point of entry and track through which the needle will pass should be infiltrated with local anaesthetic. A 16- or 18-gauge Tuohy needle is then inserted into the back, passing through skin, subcutaneous fat, supraspinous ligaments and meeting resistance at the *ligamentum flavum*. A special low-resistance syringe is attached to the needle filled with saline (or less commonly air). Continuous pressure should be applied to the plunger of the syringe whilst the needle is slowly advanced; when the needle reaches the *ligamentum flavum*, the resistance may increase. However, it is the loss of resistance to the saline in the syringe that indicates the epidural space has been found. (3 marks)

(c) Complications of an epidural include:

- *Failure* Quoted rates vary, however up to 1 in 10 epidurals require replacement or repositioning due to a unilateral or inadequate block. (1 mark)
- *Dural puncture* Rates are somewhere around 1 in 100 to 1 in 200 depending on the operator. Individual rates can be sought from the person doing the procedure. (1 mark)

- *Nerve injury* It is difficult to give a precise figure and it depends whether you are referring to a nerve injury that lasts several weeks to months (neuropraxia) or permanent neurological damage. 1 in 10,000 to 1 in 20,000 is often quoted. Remember, you should really talk about nerve damage following *childbirth* as the majority of injuries are not as a result of epidurals! Permanent paraplegia is extremely rare. (2 marks)
- *Risk of caesarean section/assisted delivery* There is no evidence to suggest that epidurals cause an increased caesarean section rate; however, parturients undergoing prolonged and difficult labours are more likely to require epidural analgesia and are also more likely to require caesarean section delivery. Rates of assisted deliveries (forceps, ventouse), on the other hand, may have a slightly increased rate. (1 mark)
- *Hypotension* A possibility with each top up with local anaesthetic. (1 mark)
- Pressure sores, epidural abscess, epidural haematoma, intravascular injection are rare but recognised complications. (1 mark)

ANSWER 8

(a) This is the cardiac catheter.
(b) The left coronary artery (left main stem).
(c) In most people (> 80%) the left coronary artery supplies
  - the left atrium
  - the left ventricle
  - the anterior septum
(d) The circumflex artery.
(e) The posterior intraventricular branch (of the circumflex artery).
(f) The left anterior descending artery (anterior intraventricular branch).
(g) The right coronary artery.
(h) The right coronary artery, left anterior descending and the circumflex (C, E and F).
(i) The right coronary artery in 60%.
(j) The right coronary artery in 80%–90%.
(k) The phrenic nerve.
(l) Parasympathetic supply is via the vagus nerve (Xth cranial nerve); the sympathetic supply is via the sympathetic outflow of T1–T4 (C1–T5).

(m)   The vagus nerves arise from three cranial nuclei on the upper medulla (dorsal nucleus of vagus, nucleus ambiguus and nucleus of the tractus solitarius). They descend in the posterolateral groove of the brainstem, passing through the jugular foramen in the carotid sheath and in front of the cervical sympathetic chain. The left vagus runs down between the subclavian and left carotid arteries, behind the brachiocephalic vein, and over the aortic arch into the thorax giving off cardiac, pulmonic and pericardial branches. As it crosses the aorta, it gives off the left recurrent laryngeal nerve. On the right, the course is in front of the right subclavian artery, behind the right innominate vein and then it descends into the thorax next to the trachea. Its further course in the chest is similar to the left.

ANSWER 9

(a)   This is a pulse oximeter that measures the saturation of haemoglobin.

(b)   The trace from a pulse oximeter can be used to assess more than just the saturation of haemoglobin. It can be used to determine the pulse rate, whether there is adequate perfusion to the finger (therefore an indirect reflection of blood pressure) and an irregular trace may indicate the presence of an arrhythmia.

(c)   A co-oximeter is a form of spectroscope. It allows differentiation of the various forms of haemoglobin (methaemoglobin, carboxyhaemoglobin, sulphaemoglobin, HbO_2 (oxyhaemoglobin), HHb (deoxyhaemoglobin)), by using four or five different wavelengths. It is an in-vitro test; the red cells are lysed to create free haemoglobin which is then exposed to visible light of varying wavelengths (usually separated by various bandwidth filters). Hence, it differs from pulse oximetry in that it is in-vitro and that it uses different (visible spectra) light.

(d)   Two different wavelengths of light are emitted by two light-emitting diodes (LEDs). These light impulses, having passed through the finger, are detected by a photo-detector. Arterial blood flows in a pulsatile manner, which is converted into an AC signal. The light absorbed by the tissues and the venous component is constant and gives rise to a DC signal. The DC signal is ignored and the AC signal amplified. The proportion of the two wavelengths absorbed gives a percentage of oxygenated to deoxygenated haemoglobin.

(e)   The device is only accurate to 70% saturation (interestingly this was the saturation level to which healthy test volunteers were allowed to drop!). Excessive ambient light, electrical interference (eg diathermy) and inadequate circulation will all lead to an inaccurate reading. (2 marks)

Pulsatile venous flow, for example in severe tricuspid regurgitation, leads to the venous component in the finger being confused with the arterial component. (1 mark)

The probe confuses substances that absorb light in a similar frequency to haemoglobin. Substances that can cause a false reading include nail polish (especially blue), carboxyhaemoglobin, methaemoglobinaemia, and dyes such as methylene blue or indocyanine green. Bilirubin, although often quoted as affecting readings, does not absorb light in the wavelengths used and therefore has no effect on pulse oximetry readings; it does affect co-oximetry readings. (3 marks)

(f)   This occurs where the blood pressure cuff is elevated on the arm which has a pulse oximeter attached.

(g)   Myoglobin is similar to haemoglobin, but only carries one molecule of oxygen. It has relatively higher affinity for oxygen however, and hence acts as a store in skeletal and cardiac muscle.

(h)   Points A are the isosbestic points at which the absorption of HHb and HbO_2 are identical. Points B and C are the emitted wavelengths of light used by the apparatus to maximise the differences in absorption (660nm red and 940nm infrared).

ANSWER 10

(a)

Group	Incidence (%)	Red cell antigen	Plasma antibodies
A	42	a	b
B	8	b	a
AB	3	a and b	none
O	47	none	a and b

(b)   Type M antibodies.

(c)   Yes. However, this should only be as a last resort. If the woman is of child-bearing age the transfusion should be accompanied by anti-D, otherwise she is at risk of developing rhesus antibodies leading to haemolytic disease of the newborn. The woman is also at risk of a transfusion reaction, if for some reason she has been previously exposed to rhesus positive blood.

(d)   This is saline, adenine, glucose and mannitol. This combination is used to resuspend washed red cells for transfusion as packed red cells.
Saline is used to suspend the red blood cells, reducing the haematocrit of the packed cells.
Adenine and glucose are both substrates to help maintain the structure and function of the red blood cell.
Mannitol is used to prevent haemolysis.

ANSWER 11

(a)   Alternating current with a frequency of 0.5–1 MHz.

(b)   Suturing (ligation of vessel), harmonic scalpel, laser and topical oxidised regenerated cellulose, absorbable haemostat, eg Surgicel®.

(c)   The patient is not electrocuted, as he or she is only exposed to a current with a high frequency. A capacitor allows the diathermy current to flow whilst preventing the flow of the more harmful 50 Hz current. The circuitry used is a floating circuit and so will be safe under single fault conditions also.

(d)   A diathermy return plate works by reducing current density by increasing the surface area through which the current flows. The surface area is of key importance; a reduction by 50% in the size of a plate will lead to a fourfold increase in the heating effect under the plate, potentially causing burns. The efficacy of the plate is also affected by how well it makes contact with the skin. Areas of vascular insufficiency, areas of the body that distribute heat poorly, eg bony prominences, or areas that may heat up abnormally, eg over a prosthesis, should be avoided. Finally, the current does not flow uniformly towards the patient plate as its density is higher at the corners and the edges of the plate *nearest* the active electrode. Therefore, the patient plate should be placed with its longest edge pointing towards the active electrode.

(e)   Muscle moves and contracts due to a local effect of heating of the tissue leading to calcium release, not as a result of electrical stimulation.

(f)   A shows a continuous sine wave employed in cutting; B, the pulsed square wave of coagulation; C, a mixture of the two or 'blend'.
(g)   Undesirable effects include:
■ Faulty equipment can lead to electrocution
■ Interference with pacemaker function, especially unipolar diathermy
■ Interference with other electrical monitoring equipment, eg ECG
■ Arcing can occur with metal instruments
■ Burns and fires can occur with spirit-based skin preparation solutions
■ Burns underneath the indifferent electrode can occur if the plate is applied incorrectly
■ Channelling effects can occur if unipolar diathermy is used on structures with a pedicle, eg testis.

ANSWER 12

(a)   Atrial fibrillation.
(b)   Causes of atrial fibrillation include ischaemic heart disease, mitral valve disease, electrolyte imbalance, thyrotoxicosis, alcohol intoxication, sepsis, hypertension, pulmonary embolism, cardiomyopathy, irritation of the myocardium by wire or cannula, pericarditis, atrial septal defect, myocarditis and sick sinus syndrome. (1/2 mark each maximum 4 total)
(c)   Drugs used primarily to control the ventricular response include β-blockers, cardiac glycosides (digoxin) and calcium antagonists. Other drugs are primarily intended to cardiovert chemically; these include Vaughan Williams class IA drugs quinidine, procainamide and disopyramide; IC flecainide and propafenone; Class III amiodarone, sotalol. If successful, these drugs will obviously have a rate-controlling effect!
(d)   β-blockers would be contraindicated due to her severe respiratory disease and flecainide would be contraindicated due to her age and cardiac history.
(e)   It does depend on the underlying cardiac function; however, it is usually reduced by about 25%–30%.
(f)   The shock should be synchronised as this avoids an R-on-T phenomenon and ventricular fibrillation occurring.
(g)   According to the Resuscitation Council Guidelines, 200 J should be used initially, increasing as required.

(h) According to the resuscitation council guidelines 120–150 J should be used initially increasing as necessary.

ANSWER 13

(a) The following foramina and contents are shown: (2 marks each)
  A *Foramen magnum* Medulla oblongata and meninges, vertebral artery and spinal accessory nerve.
  B *Hypoglossal canal* Hypoglossal nerve and meningeal branches of the ascending pharyngeal artery.
  C *Jugular foramen* Sigmoid and inferior petrosal sinuses, vagus and accessory nerves.
  D *Internal auditory meatus* Facial and vestibulocochlear nerves and labyrinthine vessels.
  E *Foramen lacerum* Small meningeal branch of the pharyngeal artery and emissary vein.
  F *Foramen spinosum* Middle meningeal vessels and meningeal branch of the mandibular nerve.
  G *Foramen ovale* Mandibular division of the trigeminal and lesser petrosal nerve.
  H *Foramen rotundum* Maxillary division of the trigeminal nerve.
  I *Optic canal* Optic nerve and ophthalmic artery.
  J *Foramen caecum* Emissary vein.

ANSWER 14

(a) Yes, the vertebral bodies are visible.
(b) Female.
(c) Multiple rib fractures and a haemothorax on the right side.
(d) Flail chest.
(e) ABCD approach should be taken. The adequacy of her ventilation should be monitored with regular blood gases and pulse oximetry. A chest drain should be inserted to drain the haemothorax. Large-bore intravenous access should be inserted and fluid resuscitation should be given. This patient may well require additional respiratory support. Adequate analgesia is essential and the patient should also be cared for in a high dependency area.
(f) A thoracic epidural.
(g) Cerebral venogram.
(h) Thrombosis in the right transverse sinus.
(i) Falx cerebri.

(j)　　The sigmoid sinus (C), the transverse sinus (E) and the straight sinus (D).

(k)　　Inferior sagittal sinus and great cerebral vein.

(l)　　The CSF is produced by the choroid plexi and it flows from the lateral ventricles to the third ventricle (via the foramina of Munro) and then to the 4th ventricle via the aqueduct of Sylvius. It then passes from the 4th ventricle through the foramina of Magendie and Luschka down the spinal cord and up over the cerebral hemispheres. Finally it is absorbed by the arachnoid villi.

ANSWER 15

(a)　　The atrial rate is 96 beats per minute (bpm), and the ventricular rate is 66 bpm. There is second-degree heart block with progressive lengthening of the PR interval followed by a lack of AV conduction. The axis is normal. There are also features of an inferior MI with ST elevation, T wave inversion and pathological Q waves in II, III, and aVF.

(b)　　Common causes of the Wenckebach phenomenon:
- Normal variant in athletes
- In conditions of increased vagal tone
- Following an inferior MI
- With drugs that reduce the AV conduction rate, eg digoxin, β-blockers

(c)　　There is no ECG evidence of any valve lesion requiring antibiotic prophylaxis.

(d)　　There is no evidence of hyperkalaemia or hypokalaemia.

(e)　　The ECG shows sinus rhythm, with a rate of 84 bpm. There is right axis deviation (+125°). Leads V_1, II, III, aVF have tall P waves (>1.5 mm) suggestive of atrial hypertrophy. There is also a dominant R wave in V_1 and deep S wave in the lateral leads suggestive of right ventricular hypertrophy.

(f)　　Congenital cardiac defects are present in about 50% of Down syndrome patients. They include (in decreasing order of frequency) AV septal defects, ventral septal defects, patent ductus arteriosus, tetralogy of Fallot (pulmonary stenosis, VSD, overriding aorta, right ventricular hypertrophy), and atrial septal defects. With the increasing life expectancy of Down syndrome patients, there is an increasing incidence of acquired cardiac disease (ischaemia and degenerative valve defects, etc).

(g)   The presence of late-onset cyanosis in Down syndrome with right-sided cardiac hypertrophy is highly suggestive of Eisenmenger syndrome.

ANSWER 16

(a)   CTG stands for cardiotocograph.
(b)   The normal range is 120–160 bpm.
(c)   The bottom trace measures uterine contractions in mmHg.
(d)   This CTG shows early decelerations, and should not be a trigger for a caesarean section. Early decelerations are commonly seen at this stage of labour; if they occur in early labour or antenatally then they are of more concern. None of this should affect your anaesthetic technique in this case. Your decision as how to proceed should be guided by the clinical status of the mother and in discussion with the obstetrician.
(e)   This shows late decelerations and is an indicator of fetal distress.
(f)   *True.*
(g)   *False.*
(h)   *True.*
(i)   *False* The left lateral position is used to relieve aorto-caval compression.
(j)   *True.*
(k)   *False* Until some years ago phenylephrine was thought to vasoconstrict utero-placental arterial flow; however, the increase in maternal blood pressure more than overcomes this and in fact flow to the placenta is improved.
(l)   *False.*
(m)   *True.*
(n)   *False.*

ANSWER 17

(a)   *False.*
(b)   *False.*
(c)   *True.*
(d)   *True.*
(e)   *False* The two treatment arms would make it two-tailed.
       Where a significant benefit has been established, it is considered unethical to deny patients the obvious benefits of a drug through randomisation, assuming the published trial is of an acceptable

standard. The new trial should be abandoned although it could be modified to use an ethical historical control.

(f)
- *Phase I* concerns healthy volunteers or fit patients. Investigations are usually carried out by a clinical pharmacologist on 50–100 subjects for the purpose of determining pharmacokinetics, pharmacodynamics, tolerance and safety. With some drugs, eg anti-cancer treatments, there may be early availability of the drug to named patients to start the efficacy studies. (3 marks)
- *Phase II* is carried out on up to 200 patients who may benefit. It is carried out by a clinical pharmacologist whose aim is to determine efficacy, dose–response and safety. It may involve a double- or single-blind trial. (3 marks)
- *Phase III* is carried out by clinicians in the specialty on patients in order to determine the efficacy and safety on a larger population. A double-blinded trial recruiting 2000–5000 patients is usually carried out. (3 marks)
- *Phase IV* again involves clinicians reporting back to provide data on use of the drug in clinical practice. This is sometime referred to as post-marketing surveillance. During this phase it is hoped that infrequent events will come to light. (3 marks)

(g)   *False* Outliers should not be removed just because they distort the correlation. They may however be investigated to determine whether an error has taken place, eg in sampling. Following the investigation a case can sometimes be made for their removal.

(h)   *True* Mathematical modification of data is acceptable, eg logarithms, in order to make data more useful.

(i)   *False* A correlation of 0.9 does suggest a strong a degree of association. However, it does not prove a causal relationship between the variables.

Structured Objective Examinations

Physiology Questions

You are shown these arterial blood gas results:

pH 7.22, PCO_2 2.4 kPa, PO_2 15.5 kPa, HCO_3 7.7 mmol/l, base deficit −19.1

    What is the normal acid–base status and why is it important?
    What does this arterial blood gas indicate?
    What is the differential diagnosis?
    What do you understand by the anion gap?
    How does the body compensate for the acidosis?
    Define what a buffer is. What are the buffer systems?
    Buffers accept or donate H^+ ions in order to try to maintain normal pH.
    What is pH?
    What is the difference between acidosis and acidaemia?
    What is a nanomol?
    Is it possible to have a PO_2 of 15.5 kPa whilst breathing room air at sea level?
    What do you understand by the term minute ventilation?
    By what mechanisms does the PCO_2 affect respiration?

2

    What is the Fick principle?
    What applications of the Fick principle are you aware of?
    Talk me through how the Fick principle can be used to calculate cardiac output.

3

    What is the role of the hypothalamus?
    How do we regulate our temperature?
    What factors can disturb thermoregulation?

Define hypothermia. What are the causes of hypothermia?
What are the physiological effects of hypothermia?
Why does anaesthesia cause hypothermia?
What are the routes of heat loss during surgery and anaesthesia?
How can heat loss be prevented during surgery and anaesthesia?
What are the problems associated with intraoperative hypothermia?

4

What do you understand by the term basal metabolic rate (BMR)?
What is the energy required for?
What factors influence BMR?
How can BMR be measured?
What factors influence the ratio of CO_2 produced to O_2 consumed?
In the early stages of anaerobic exercise what would you expect the RQ to be?
How does the RQ change in chronic respiratory disease? How can we influence this with diet?

5

What do you understand by the cardiac cycle?
Draw a graph to show the cardiac cycle and relate it to electrical activity in the heart. Explain what the graph tells us and what is happening.
Where does the mitral valve open?
Where does the aortic valve close?
What are the functions of diastole?
Draw a loop that relates pressure to volume in a normal left ventricle.
How do you calculate the stroke volume from this loop?
What is the normal stroke volume?
What factors affect the stroke volume?
How do you use the stroke volume to calculate the ejection fraction?
What is the normal ejection fraction?
What does the area of the loop correspond to?
How can the loop be used to assess diastolic function?
How would this curve look in a hypertrophied heart?
What are the three peaks that you see in an atrial pressure curve?
Can you draw and explain the atrial waveform?

6

What are the main reasons for giving fluid to patients in the peri-operative period?

What are the basic adult maintenance requirements?

How much water is there in the average 70-kg man?

How is this divided into various body compartments?

How does knowledge of the composition of fluid compartments affect our choice of fluids to give to a patient who has lost extracellular fluid?

What is the difference between NSaline and compound sodium lactate?

Why is there lactate in Hartmanns?

What do you understand by the term isotonic?

Which fluids that we use are isotonic?

What is the difference between osmolality and osmolarity?

Why are these terms sometimes used interchangeably when referring to body fluids?

What is the normal osmolality of plasma and how is it maintained?

What do we mean by the term hypotonic fluids?

When would you use hypotonic fluids? What are the problems associated with their use?

What are colloids? Give some examples. What are the problems associated with their use?

7

What is the role of the autonomic nervous system?

Tell me about the parasympathetic nervous system. Which nerves does it involve and what ganglia do the nerves pass through? Where does each nerve terminate? What is the neurotransmitter?

Tell me about the sympathetic nervous system and the nerves that it involves.

8

What is a spirometer?

Draw a spirometer trace of the lung volumes.

What is the vital capacity?

What factors affect vital capacity?

When is it important to measure vital capacity?

What is the functional residual capacity?

Can FRC be measured using spiromtery?

How can FRC be derived?
What is the closing capacity?
Define FEV$_1$ and FVC.
Why is the FVC different from the vital capacity?
Draw a graph to indicate their relationship and how this changes in disease.
How will a flow volume loop change with obstructive and restrictive lung disease?

9

What is the blood supply to the heart?
What is the normal coronary blood flow?
Why is coronary blood flow unique?
What factors determine coronary blood flow?
How can coronary blood flow be measured?

10

Draw the oxygen dissociation curve.
What factors move it to the left and right?
Why is the curve sigmoid in shape?
What is the Bohr effect?
What is the Haldane effect?
What compensatory changes due to hypoxia occur at high altitude?
What effect do these compensatory changes have on the oxygen dissociation curve?
Why is the oxyhaemoglobin curve relevant in pregnancy?

Pharmacology Questions

1

What is a local anaesthetic agent and how does it work?
How are local anaesthetics classified?
What are the recommended doses of lignocaine and bupivacaine?
Why does bupivacaine work more slowly than lignocaine?
What role does the racemic mixture play in the problem of bupivacaine toxicity?
In what way does inflammation affect local anaesthetic efficacy? Why?
What characteristics of local anaesthetics affect their onset of action, potency and duration of action?

2

What are the uses of non-steroidal anti-inflammatory drugs (NSAIDs)?
How do NSAIDs work?
Draw the pathway that they interrupt.
What are the side-effects of NSAIDs? How can we avoid them?
In which situations would you avoid giving patients NSAIDs?
Give some examples of selective NSAIDs.
How does aspirin differ from other NSAIDs?
What are the features of an aspirin overdose? How can the overdose be treated?

3

What factors affect the uptake of anaesthetic agents from inhaled gas into the blood?
Draw a graph to indicate the relationship between the alveolar concentration and inspired concentration of a gas and the wash in times for different volatile agents.
What does the graph tell you about the solubility of the gas with the F_A/F_I closest to 1?
Why is saturated vapour pressure (SVP) important? What is the SVP of desflurane?
What does the oil gas coefficient indicate?
How is it relevant to how anaesthetics are believed to work?
Draw a graph of MAC versus oil gas coefficient and plot the main volatile agents.

What are the advantages and disadvantages of using desflurane?
Compare the physical properties of desflurane and sevoflurane.
Draw the structure of sevoflurane and desflurane.
What are the problems associated with sevoflurane metabolism?

4

What is an inotrope?
What is the difference between an inotrope and a vasopressor?
Classify inotropes.
Discuss dopexamine.
In what situations do we give adrenaline?
What are the routes by which adrenaline can be given?
What effect does adrenaline have on systemic vascular resistance?
What dose and concentration of adrenaline would you give for the treatment of anaphylaxis?
What is the rationale for use of adrenaline in CPR

5

If I take this beaker of water, pretend it is a patient's blood and add my drug A to it, how do I calculate the volume of distribution of the drug?
Let us assume a one-compartment model. What will happen to the concentration of the drug over time? Draw a graph to represent this. How can we make this graph easier to interpret?
How can we calculate the clearance?
How can we calculate the half-life?
What do you understand by the context sensitive half-life?
What are the drawbacks of pharmacokinetic models?

6

What types of neuromuscular blocking drugs are there?
How do their mechanisms of action differ?
What can happen if you give a second dose of suxamethonium?
What are the advantages of rocuronium?
What are the properties of an ideal neuromuscular blocker?

7

What do we use benzodiazepines for in clinical practice?
What is the mechanism of action of benzodiazepines?
Why is temazepam preferred for night-time sedation compared with diazepam?
Compare midazolam and diazepam.
What kind of isomerism does midazolam display?
How are benzodiazepines metabolised?
What are the principles of treating benzodiazepine poisoning?

8

What is an adverse drug reaction?
What is the term we use to describe a genetically determined adverse drug reaction?
Give some examples of idiosyncratic drug reactions.
Expand on the mechanism of idiosyncrasy in these examples.
By what process would you manage and report a suspected adverse drug reaction?
What does this symbol mean when next to a drug in the *British National Formulary*?

9

Name some drugs that are known to cause emesis.
Explain the various neural inputs that result in vomiting.
What neurotransmitters are involved in nausea and vomiting?
What anti-emetics do you know of? What is their mode of action?
How can we administer anti-emetics?
Name any drugs that can be administered transdermally.

10

What is a dose–response curve?

Draw a curve to indicate a competitive reversible antagonist and one to indicate a competitive irreversible antagonist. Give examples of such drugs.

Give an example of non-competitive antagonism.

What are partial agonists? Draw a curve to indicate the response. Give an example.

What is an inverse agonist? Draw a graph to indicate the response.

Physics and Clinical Measurement Questions

1

What do you understand by the Venturi effect?

What is the Bernoulli principle?

How does a Venturi mask use these principles to deliver different oxygen concentrations?

What is the entrainment ratio?

What is the usual entrainment ratio in Venturi masks?

What are the other uses of Venturi?

If Venturi masks are fixed performance devices, give an example of a variable performance device. What factors will affect the final F_iO_2 in a variable performance device?

What is the Coanda effect?

2

Define humidity.

What are the normal values for humidity in the upper trachea and the alveoli?

How can we measure humidity? Describe how each method works.

What is the humidity achievable by heat and moisture exchange filtration (HMEF)?

What is the normal operating theatre humidity? What are the risks in theatre if the humidity is too low?

3

What methods are used to measure volatile gases? Which is the most common in a modern anaesthetic machine? Describe how each method works.

How do we measure oxygen?

Tell me how the Clark electrode works.

4

What is ultrasound?

What is the Doppler effect/shift?

Why is the Doppler effect relevant to us?

Give some examples of how the Doppler is used clinically.

5

What is a pulse oximeter?
How does it work?
How does the pulse oximeter compensate for ambient light?
What can lead to inaccuracies in the pulse oximeter reading?
What are the risks with pulse oximeter use?
What monitors do you consider essential to the safe conduct of anaesthesia?

6

What do you understand by the term flow?
What is the difference between laminar and turbulent flow?
What equations do you know that explain the different types of flow?
What is the Reynolds' number?
What is the critical velocity?
What devices do we use to measure flow? How can we classify them?
What is a rotameter?
Where do you read the gas flow from when you have a bobbin or a ball?
In which positions will a rotameter function?
What safety features are employed in flowmeters?

7

Here are photos of measuring devices. What do they measure? Name each type of instrument and describe how it works.

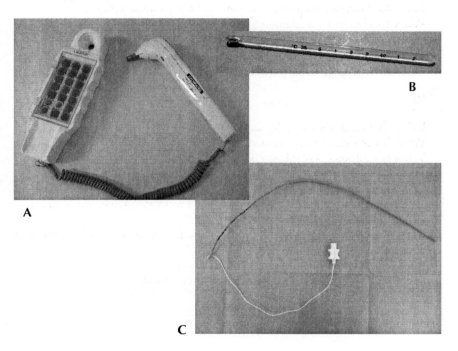

A

B

C

How can we classify the ways in which temperature is measured?
How does a thermocouple work?
Where can temperature be measured?
Where can you get an accurate core temperature reading?
What are the temperature scales that you know of? Tell me about them.

8

What types of breathing system do you know of?
Draw the outline of a circle breathing system.
What is low-flow anaesthesia?
What are the advantages and disadvantages of low-flow anaesthesia?

9

What is diathermy? What types of diathermy do you know of?
When is unipolar diathermy used and when is bipolar diathermy used?
Why does diathermy not affect the cardiac and skeletal muscle?
You are shown two plates (one for a child, one for an adult). Where should the plate be placed and why? Discuss the current density.
What is a capacitor?
Why is there a capacitor in the diathermy circuit?
What are the hazards associated with diathermy?
Name the following electrical symbols.

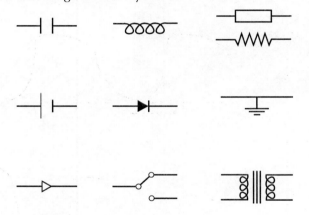

10

How do we measure CO_2?

Tell me how the infrared analyser works.

What is collision broadening and how do we prevent it causing reading errors?

What types of capnograph are there?

What do the following capnograph traces indicate?

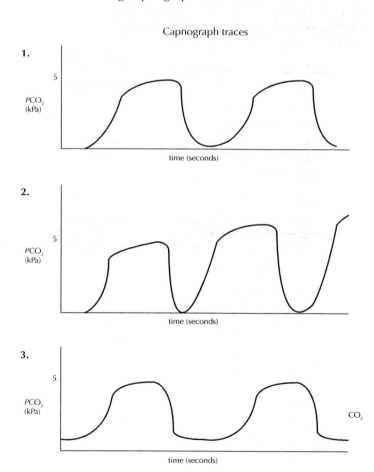

Capnograph traces

Clinical Questions

A 60-year-old woman with asthma for emergency repair of detached retina.

How would you assess an asthmatic preoperatively?
How would you treat a severe asthmatic?
What are the side-effects of salbutamol if used in high doses?
Which is more important to continue, the β-agonist or steroids?
Is a CXR an important investigation in this scenario?
How would you anaesthetise this patient?
What is your postoperative care for a severe asthmatic?

Critical incident: there is a sudden increase in airway pressures.
What is your approach to this situation?

When you auscultate the chest you discover there is severe bronchospasm
What action will you take?

On further auscultation you discover that there is hyper-resonance and absent breath sounds on the right-hand side of the chest
What is your diagnosis and what will you do?
What are the causes of a pneumothorax in the perioperative period that could be caused by the anaesthetist?

2

Do you give blood to your patients? Do you discuss this with them preoperatively?
What happens when you ask for the blood to be group and saved?
Tell me about the ABO blood group system.
What happens when you ask for blood to be cross matched?
What types of blood are available to you when you need to give a blood transfusion?

Here is an empty blood bag. Go through what you would do to check the blood.

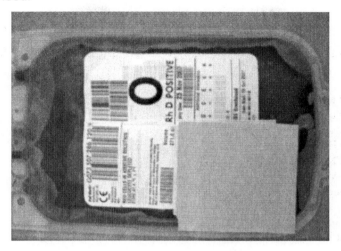

How is blood stored?
What is autologous blood transfusion?
Why is blood leucodepleted?
What is the definition of a massive blood transfusion?
What is your management of a massive blood loss?
What problems are associated with blood transfusion?

3

You are the SHO on call in a busy District General Hospital. You are asked to anaesthetise an 8-year-old child for manipulation under anaesthetic (MUA) + K wire of radius.
What are the main issues in your preoperative assessment?
What should you have a high index of suspicion for in any child with a fracture?
If the weight of the child was not available how could you approximate the weight?
How will you anaesthetise this child?
What size LMA and what size tube would you use?
How would you calculate how much fluid to give the child if you were just giving maintenance fluids?

During the procedure you notice the carbon dioxide is rising rapidly and the child is tachycardic.

What do you do?

What are the triggers for malignant hyperthermia?

What is the genetic explanation for malignant hyperthermia?

You are asked to anaesthetise an 87-year-old man for transurethral resection of the prostate (TURP).

What are the potential problems?

You opt for a spinal anaesthetic for the procedure

What risks do you tell the patient about?

What kind of spinal needle would you use and why?

What drugs would you give via the spinal route?

Towards the end of the procedure the patient becomes agitated, restless and confused

What will you do?

What is TURP syndrome?

How can TURP syndrome be avoided?

Structured Objective Examinations — Answers

Physiology Answers

You are shown these arterial blood gas results:

pH 7.22, PCO_2 2.4 kPa, PO_2 15.5 kPa, HCO_3 7.7 mmol/l, base deficit −19.1

What is the normal acid–base status and why is it important?
Normal acid–base status comprises a pH of 7.34–7.46, a plasma HCO_3 of 25 mmol/l and a PCO_2 of 5.5 kPa.

A stable pH is necessary for normal enzyme activity, ion distribution and protein structure and function.

Top tip
Get used to using kPa rather than mmHg
To convert mmHg to kPa just divide by 7.5

What does this arterial blood gas indicate?
There is a metabolic acidosis with respiratory compensation.

We can tell there is a metabolic acidosis by the low bicarbonate and negative base deficit.

What is the differential diagnosis?
Causes of a metabolic acidosis are due to:

Increased acid
- ↑ Acid production: ketone bodies, lactacte
- ↑ Acid ingestion: salicylate poisoning
- ↓ Acid excretion: failure to excrete H^+ ions; renal failure, renal tubular acidosis, carbonic anhydrase inhibitors

Loss of bicarbonate
>   Diarrhoea, GI fistulae, proximal renal tubular acidosis, ureter enter-
>   oscopy.

What do you understand by the anion gap?

The anion gap can be helpful in distinguishing the cause of the acidosis. It measures the difference between the cations and anions in the plasma. An increased gap usually means that bicarbonate is being used to titrate excess acid, and usually reflects a metabolic acidosis. Lactic acidosis is a normal 'anion-gap' acidosis.

$$\text{anion gap} = [Na^+]+[K^+]-[Cl^-]+[HCO_3^-]$$

The normal anion gap is between 8 and 12 units.

How does the body compensate for the acidosis?

Buffer systems work within seconds, the respiratory system acts within minutes and the renal system works within hours to try to restore normal pH.

The respiratory response is hyperventilation and this is why the CO_2 is low. As the acidosis becomes more severe Kussmaul breathing or 'air hunger' can develop. The kidneys will compensate with increased H^+ secretion, decreased HCO_3 loss.

Define what a buffer is. What are the buffer systems?

Bicarbonate buffer – Henderson–Hasselbalch equation
Phosphate buffers
Protein buffers, eg albumin, haemoglobin.

Buffers accept or donate H^+ ions in order to try to maintain normal pH. What is pH?

pH is the negative logarithm to the base 10 of hydrogen ion concentration.

$$pH=-\log_{10}[H^+]$$

pH	[H⁺] (nmol/l)
7.0	100
7.3	50
7.6	25

What is the difference between acidosis and acidaemia?
Acidemia is an arterial pH<7.35.
Acidosis is a process in which arterial pH is < 7.35 or would be <7.35 if there were no compensatory mechanisms.

What is a nanomol?
1 nanomol = 10^{-9} mol per litre.

Is it possible to have a PO_2 of 15.5 kPa whilst breathing room air at sea level?
It is possible in the presence of hyperventilation when the P_aCO_2 is low.

We can work this out by using the alveolar gas equation given by $P_aO_2 = P_iO_2 - P_aCO_2 /R + F$, where R is the respiratory exchange ratio, normally 0.8, and F is a correction factor.

If $P_iO_2=(PB-PH_2O) \times F_iO_2$, where PB =101.3 kPa and PH_2O=6.3 kPa, then $P_iO_2=(101.3-6.3) \times 0.21= 19.95$ kPa

$P_aCO_2=19.95-2.3/0.8=17.07$ kPa

What do you understand by the term minute ventilation?
It is the volume of air breathed per minute (= tidal volume × respiratory rate). The normal minute ventilation is 5–7 l/min or 6–10 ml/kg per min.

By what mechanisms does the PCO_2 affect respiration?
Via peripheral and central chemoreceptors.

Peripheral chemoreceptors respond to changes in PCO_2 and pH via the aortic bodies (via CN X) and carotid bodies (via CN IX).

Central chemoreceptors in the ventral medulla respond to H^+ changes as CO_2 diffuses over the blood–brain barrier.

These both input into the respiratory centre in the medulla which initiates a change in minute volume.

2

What is the Fick principle?

The blood flow to an organ/unit time is equal to the amount of marker substance taken up by the organ in that time divided by the concentration difference of the substance in the vessels supplying and draining the organ.

What applications of the Fick principle are you aware of?

There are a number of applications of the Fick principle:
1. Blood flow
   a. Cerebral blood flow: Kety Schmidt technique using N_2O
   b. Renal blood flow using *para*-aminohippuric acid (PAH)
   c. Coronary blood flow using N_2O or argon
2. Cardiac output
   a. O_2
   b. CO_2.

Talk me through how the Fick principle can be used to calculate cardiac output.

Cardiac output$=O_2$ consumption$/(C_aO_2-C_vO_2)$
    $=250$ ml/min divided by $(200-150)$ ml/l
    $=5$ l/min

or

Cardiac output$= CO_2$ output$/(C_vCO_2-C_aCO_2)$
    $= 200$ ml/min divided by $(540-500)$ ml/l
    $= 5$ l/min

3

What is the role of the hypothalamus?

The hypothalamus is a regulation centre that controls autonomic functions and hormonal output from the anterior pituitary.

Autonomic functions regulated by the hypothalamus include cardiovascular and temperature regulation along with feeding, sexual behaviour and water balance.

How do we regulate our temperature?
Heat loss responses
>Behavioural: remove clothes, go outside
>Cutaneous vasodilatation
>Sweating
>Panting

Heat gain responses
>Behavioural: put on clothes, turn up the heat
>Exercise
>Cutaneous vasoconstriction
>Shivering
>Non-shivering thermogenesis.

What factors can disturb thermoregulation?
Fever
Malignant hyperthermia
Hypothermia
Anaesthesia.

Define hypothermia. What are the causes of hypothermia?
Hypothermia is said to be present when core body temperature is less than 36°C.

Hypothermia can be associated with exposure, near drowning, the elderly, hypothyroidism, anaesthesia and prolonged surgery.

What are the physiological effects of hypothermia?
Metabolic and physiological processes may be slowed down leading to hypotension, bradycardia, bradypnoea and loss of consciousness developing into pulmonary oedema and ventricular fibrillation in severe cases.

Why does anaesthesia cause hypothermia?
Loss of behavioural responses.
Greater area of patient exposed to atmosphere with rapid air movement due to ventilation.
Cutaneous vasoconstriction is antagonised by vasodilator anaesthetics.
Thermoregulatory centre is depressed.

What are the routes of heat loss during surgery and anaesthesia?
There are four principle routes of heat loss from the patient.

Route	Percentage	Explanation
Radiation	40%	Heat loss by infrared radiation. Rate of heat loss depends on the relative temperatures between the patient and surrounding objects.
Convection	30%	Air layer around body warmed by conduction and as the air warms it is carried away by convection.
Evaporation	20%	Latent heat of vaporisation causes heat loss as fluid changes from liquid to vapour.
Respiration	10%	8% by increasing the humidity of inspired air and 2% due to warming of the air.

How can heat loss be prevented during surgery and anaesthesia?
Warm environment
Reduce body surface exposure
Blankets
Forced air warming blankets: Bair Hugger
Warming mattresses
Warming fluids especially blood
Insulated patient clothing: jackets, hats, leggings and outfits
Warm anaesthetic gases (use of HME device).

What are the problems associated with intraoperative hypothermia?
Increased morbidity, hypoxia, myocardial ischaemia, arrhythmias and cerebral ischaemia
Decreased drug metabolism and prolonged duration of action
Shivering and increased oxygen requirements
Coagulopathy
Increased incidence of wound breakdown and infection.

What do you understand by the term basal metabolic rate (BMR)?
The BMR is the amount of energy liberated by catabolism of food per unit time, under standardised conditions, ie a relaxed subject at comfortable temperature, 12–14 hours after a meal, corrected for age, sex and surface area. The normal BMR in an adult male is 197 kJ/m^2 per h.

What is the energy required for?
The chemical energy of food is transformed to heat even when no external work is done. This heat is used to maintain the normal bodily functions.

What factors influence BMR?
Body size: height, weight and body surface area
Sex
Age
After food: specific dynamic action
Exercise
Genetics
Environmental temperature
Growth
Hormones such as thyroxine and adrenaline
Pregnancy and lactation
Emotional state.

How can BMR be measured?

Direct calorimetry
HEAT PRODUCED: Heat produced by the subject in an insulated room whose outside walls are maintained at constant temperature. The heat produced raises the temperature of water passing through coils in the ceiling allowing calculation of BMR.

Indirect calorimetry
OXYGEN CONSUMPTION: Benedict–Roth spirometer (the volume of oxygen consumed is recorded), Douglas bag (the expired air is analysed for O_2 and CO_2 content).

What factors influence the ratio of CO_2 produced to O_2 consumed?
The concept of respiratory quotient (RQ) is used to express the ratio of the volume of CO_2 produced by tissues to the volume of O_2 consumed per unit time in steady state. A similar term is the respiratory exchange ratio (RER), when RQ is derived from expired CO_2/inspired O_2 at any given time (equilibrium may not have been reached).

It can be influenced by metabolic and non-metabolic factors.

Metabolic factors
Food substrate: glucose RQ 1, protein RQ 0.8, fat RQ 0.7
Hyperventilation:
> Exercise: during exercise the RQ approaches a value of 2
> Metabolic acidosis: the RQ increases to compensate for acidosis

Non-metabolic factors
Drugs: eg fentanyl, causes hypoventilation and therefore decreased CO_2 and reduced RQ.

In the early stages of anaerobic exercise what would you expect the RQ to be?
Since glycogen in the early stages of anaerobic exercise is the substrate I would expect it to be near to 1.

How does the RQ change in chronic respiratory disease? How can we influence this with diet?
Patients with chronic obstructive pulmonary disease (COPD) are often hypermetabolic because of their increased work of breathing, leading to an increased RQ. In COPD the amount of CO_2 retained increases, leading to acidosis which also increases the RQ. This is why in theory the diet of COPD patients can be modified to have a higher lipid content, which has a lower ratio of CO_2 production to O_2 consumed. However, it should be balanced with the fact that malnutrition can lead to muscle loss, specifically of respiratory muscles which are needed.

5

What do you understand by the cardiac cycle?
The cardiac cycle consists of a period of relaxation (diastole) followed by ventricular contraction (systole). During diastole the ventricles are relaxed to allow filling. In systole the right and left ventricles contract, ejecting blood into the pulmonary (low-resistance) and systemic circulations.

Draw a graph to show the cardiac cycle and relate it to electrical activity in the heart. Explain what the graph tells us and what is happening.

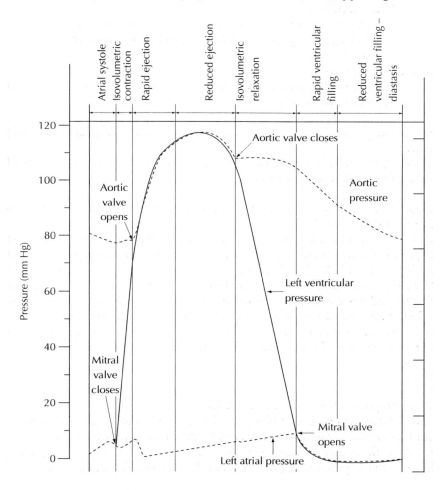

Diagram 1: Draw a graph showing LV pressure, aortic pressure, atrial pressure. Point out the phases of isovolumetric contraction and relaxation.

The pressure in the left ventricle increases during isovolumetric contraction and exceeds the pressure in the aorta. At this point the aortic valve opens and ejection begins. Ejection continues for as long as ventricular pressure exceeds the aortic pressure.

Where does the mitral valve open?

Where does the aortic valve close?

What are the functions of diastole?
Myocardial relaxation: a metabolically active phase since reuptake of calcium occurs.
Rapid ventricular filling: ventricular filling.
Slow ventricular filling
Atrial contraction
Coronary artery perfusion: the greater part of left coronary blood flow occurs during diastole.

Draw a loop that relates pressure to volume in a normal left ventricle.

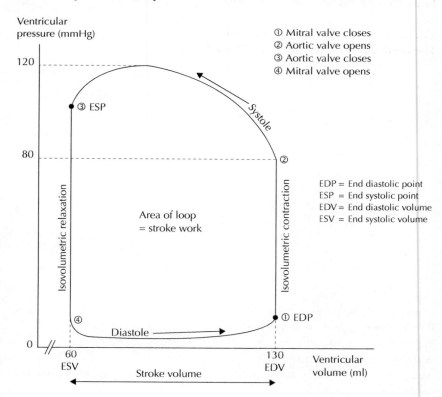

① Mitral valve closes
② Aortic valve opens
③ Aortic valve closes
④ Mitral valve opens

EDP = End diastolic point
ESP = End systolic point
EDV = End diastolic volume
ESV = End systolic volume

Diagram 2

How do you calculate the stroke volume from this loop?
The difference between end-diastolic volume (EDV) and end-systolic volume (ESV):
SV=EDV–ESV

What is the normal stroke volume?
70–80 ml

What factors affect the stroke volume?
Preload
Contractility
Systemic vascular resistance

How do you use the stroke volume to calculate the ejection fraction (EF)?
EF=SV/EDV×100

What is the normal ejection fraction?
The normal ejection fraction is 60%–65%.

What does the area of the loop correspond to?
How can the loop be used to assess diastolic function?

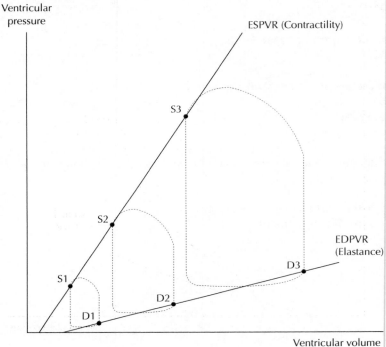

Diagram 3: End-diastolic pressure–volume relationship (EDPVR).

The steeper the gradient the lower the compliance of the ventricle during filling.

How would this curve look in a hypertrophied heart?

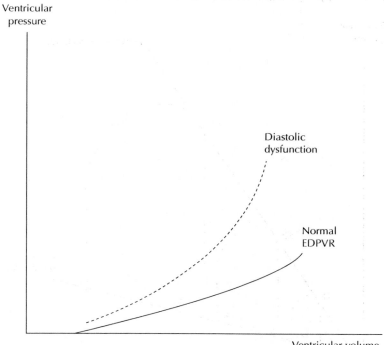

Diagram 4: Decreased compliance, sharp upturn of pressure with minimal increase in volume.

What are the three peaks that you see in an atrial pressure curve? Can you draw and explain the atrial waveform?

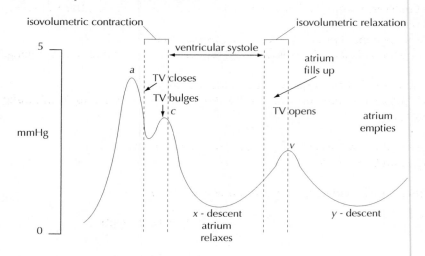

a = atrial contraction
c = bulging TV into right a during isovolumetric contraction
x = atrial relaxation
v = atrial filling (during ventricular systole)
y = atrial emptying

Contraction against a closed TV eg. CHB = Cannon *a* waves
Triscupid Regurgitation = Giant *v* waves

Diagram 5: The three peaks are the a, c and v waves.
a – atrial contraction
c – isovolumetric contraction and the AV valves (mitral and tricuspid valves) bulge back into the atrium
v – as blood is ejected from the ventricle during systole the atrium continues to fill with the AV valves closed and atrial pressure increases until early diastole when the AV valves open.

6

What are the main reasons for giving fluid to patients in the peri-operative period?
Resuscitation
Maintenance
Preparation for surgery (nil by mouth, NBM) – what is NBM time?

Bowel preparation

Replacement of ongoing losses: secondary to pyrexia, evaporative losses, NG losses, vomiting, diarrhoea, 3rd space losses, bleeding, burns, ascites, diuretics

Replacement of protracted losses, eg fistula, NG tube

Correction of electrolyte disturbances especially after diarrhoea and vomiting.

What are the basic adult maintenance requirements?
35 ml/kg per day of water with 2 mmol/kg sodium and 1 mmol/kg potassium.

How much water is there in the average 70-kg man?
42 l and 60% of body mass.

How is this divided into various body compartments?

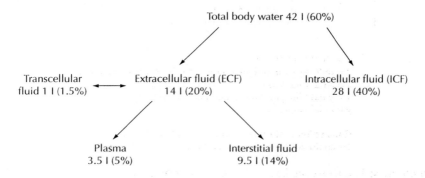

How does knowledge of the composition of fluid compartments affect our choice of fluids to give to a patient who has lost extracellular fluid?
The ionic composition of the extracellular fluid (consisting of primarily plasma and interstitial fluid) influences our choice of fluid as it contains (in mmol/l) sodium (140), potassium (5), bicarbonate (30), chloride (110), calcium (5), along with small amounts of other ions. Therefore, it is matched most physiologically to Hartmanns – compound sodium lactate (CSL) solution.

What is the difference between NSaline and compound sodium lactate?
CSL, also known as Hartmanns or Ringer's lactate, contains less sodium chloride than NSaline but contains other ions such as calcium, magnesium and bicarbonate.

	NSaline	CSL
Na	154 mmol/l	131 mmol/l
Cl	154 mmol/l	111 mmol/l
K		5 mmol/l
Calcium		2 mmol/l
Lactate		29 mmol/l
Osmolality	308 mosmol/l	279 mosmol/l
pH	5	6.5

Why is there lactate in Hartmanns?
The lactate is metabolised to bicarbonate by gluconeogenesis in the liver which avoids the hazards of giving bicarbonate.

What do you understand by the term isotonic?
Isotonic literally translates to *equal solution*. It means that the solution has the same tonicity and so exerts an equal osmotic force as plasma, which means there is no net flow of water from one solution to the other. An isotonic solution has an equal amount of dissolved solute in it compared to blood. Cells placed in an isotonic solution will not change in volume.
Tonicity describes the relative osmolality between fluid compartments.

Which fluids that we use are isotonic?
Fluids which are isotonic include normal saline 0.9%, compound sodium lactate and colloids.

What is the difference between osmolality and osmolarity?
Osmolality is the number of osmoles per kilogram solvent.
Osmolarity is the number of osmoles per litre solution.

Why are these terms sometimes used interchangeably when referring to body fluids?
In the body the solvent is water which has a density of 1 kg/l. However, proteins and fats in the plasma do give rise to a small difference.

What is the normal osmolality of plasma and how is it maintained?
The normal osmolality is maintained at 280–305 mosmol/kg. Regulatory mechanisms include thirst stimulation by osmoreceptors, baroreceptors and the renin–angiotensin system.

What do we mean by the term hypotonic fluids?

Hypotonic fluids exert a lower osmotic force than plasma. This is either because the concentration of solutes is less than in plasma or because the solute is metabolised in the plasma creating free water, which is able to move into the cells. Examples of hypotonic fluids are 0.45% NSaline and 5% dextrose.

When would you use hypotonic fluids? What are the problems associated with their use?

Hypotonic fluids such as 5% dextrose are used in paediatrics especially in neonates and in the treatment of hypoglycaemia. The main problem with hypotonic fluids is that they can lead to hyponatraemia and water overload so they should be prescribed with caution.

What are colloids? Give some examples. What are the problems associated with their use?

Colloids contain larger molecules that stay intravascularly for longer than crystalloids and exert a colloid oncotic pressure (COP). The length of time they stay in the circulation depends on the fluid. See below:

Examples are:

Colloid		Time stays in circulation (h)
Blood products	Blood or albumin 4.5% or 20%	>24
Starches	Hespan-Hetastarch mol. wt. 200 kDa Voluven mol. wt. 130 kDa	>24
Gelatins	Urea cross-linked – Haemaccel mol. wt. 30 kDa Succinylated – Gelofusin mol. wt. 30 kDa	6 2–4
Dextrans	Glucose polymer either mol. wt. 40–70 kDa	Depends on mol. wt.

There are various problems associated with colloid use:

	Interferes with blood cross match	Interferes with platelet function/ coagulation	Allergic reactions	Associated with renal failure
Blood products	Y	Y	Y	Y – with trans-fusion reaction
Starches	N	Y – slight	Y – low risk with Voluven	N
Gelatins		Y	Y	Y – Haemaccel
Dextrans	Y	Y	Y	Y

7

What is the role of the autonomic nervous system?
The autonomic nervous system regulates involuntary body functions via reflexes. It is divided into parasympathetic and sympathetic nervous systems on the basis of anatomical, pharmacological and functional differences.

Tell me about the parasympathetic nervous system. Which nerves does it involve and what ganglia do the nerves pass through? Where does each nerve terminate? What is the neurotransmitter?

Tell me about the sympathetic nervous system and the nerves that it involves.

	Parasympathetic	Sympathetic
Role	'Vegetative' Pupillary constriction ↓ CVS activity ↑ peristalsis Vasodilatation	'Fight or flight' Pupillary dilation +ve inotropy, chronotropy ↓ peristalsis Vasoconstriction
Nerves	Craniosacral III,VII,IX,X and sacral S2–S4	T1–L2, thoracolumbar outflow with sympathetic chain
Fibres	Long preganglionic and short postganglionic	Short preganglionic and long postganglionic
Neurotrans-mitters	Acetylcholine (ACh)	ACh preganglionic and noradrenaline or ACh (sweat glands) postganglionic

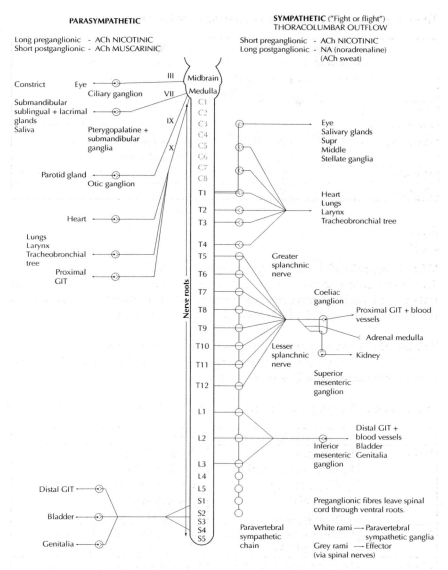

Diagram 6: Autonomic nervous system indicating nerve roots, ganglia and effector site for sympathetic vs parasympathetic systems.

8

What is a spirometer?
It is a device used for measuring lung volumes.
There are two types: the wet spirometer and the dry spirometer.

The wet spirometer consists of a cylinder suspended over a breathing chamber with a water seal. Vertical movement of the cylinder, which corresponds to respiratory movements, is recorded on a rotating drum via a pen attached to a cylinder.

The dry spirometer, like the vitalograph, contains bellows attached to a pen with a sheet of recording paper automatically moved by a motor during expiration.

Draw a spirometer trace of the lung volumes.

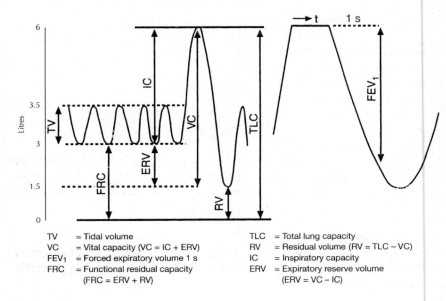

TV	= Tidal volume	TLC	= Total lung capacity	
VC	= Vital capacity (VC = IC + ERV)	RV	= Residual volume (RV = TLC – VC)	
FEV$_1$	= Forced expiratory volume 1 s	IC	= Inspiratory capacity	
FRC	= Functional residual capacity	ERV	= Expiratory reserve volume	
	(FRC = ERV + RV)		(ERV = VC – IC)	

Diagram 7

What is the vital capacity?
The vital capacity is the maximal volume of gas which can be expelled after a maximal inspiration.

What factors affect vital capacity?
Body size
Strength of respiratory muscles
Chest and lung compliance.

When is it important to measure vital capacity?
It is an important measure of respiratory sufficiency especially in restrictive diseases. Vital capacity <10 ml/kg is indicative of impending respiratory failure.

What is the functional residual capacity?
FRC is the lung volume at the end of normal expiration.
FRC=ERV +RV, where ERV is expiratory reserve volume and RV is residual volume.

Can FRC be measured using spiromtery?
Spirometry does not measure FRC and therefore RV and total lung capacity (TLC).
See diagram above.

How can FRC be derived?
FRC can be derived by:
> Helium dilution
> Body plethysmography
> Nitrogen washout.

What is the closing capacity?
The closing capacity (CC) is the closing volume plus the residual volume. It is the volume at which airway closure and collapse occur during expiration. It is important in relation to FRC. Normally CC<FRC and thus airway closure does not occur during normal breathing.

Define FEV_1 and FVC.
The FEV_1 is the volume expired in the first second and FVC is the forced vital capacity and is the total volume of gas that can be forcibly expired after maximal inspiration.

Why is the FVC different from the vital capacity?
During a forced manoeuvre there is dynamic compression of the intrathoracic airways.

Draw a graph to indicate their relationship and how this changes in disease.

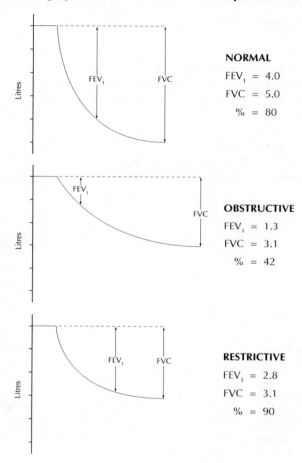

NORMAL
FEV$_1$ = 4.0
FVC = 5.0
% = 80

OBSTRUCTIVE
FEV$_1$ = 1.3
FVC = 3.1
% = 42

RESTRICTIVE
FEV$_1$ = 2.8
FVC = 3.1
% = 90

Diagram 8 The ratio indicates whether there is an obstructive or restrictive pattern of disease.

How will a flow volume loop change with obstructive and restrictive lung disease?

Normal flow volume loop
Obstructive flow volume loop
Restrictive flow volume loop

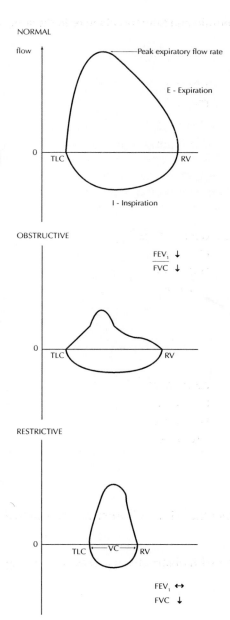

NORMAL

flow

Peak expiratory flow rate

E - Expiration

0

TLC   RV

I - Inspiration

OBSTRUCTIVE

$\dfrac{FEV_1}{FVC}$ ↓

0

TLC   RV

RESTRICTIVE

0

TLC —VC— RV

FEV_1 ↔

FVC ↓

Diagram 9

9

What is the blood supply to the heart?
The heart receives arterial blood from the left (divides into left anterior descending and circumflex branches) and right coronary arteries.

The left coronary artery arises from the left posterior aortic sinus to pass between the pulmonary trunk and left atrium into the left coronary sulcus.

The right coronary artery arises from the anterior aortic sinus before passing between the pulmonary trunk and the right atrium to run along the right coronary sulcus to anastomose with the left coronary artery.

What is the normal coronary blood flow?
250 ml/min

Why is coronary blood flow unique?
There is interruption of left coronary arterial flow during systole due to mechanical compression of vessels by myocardial contraction. Coronary blood flow occurs predominantly during diastole when cardiac muscle relaxes and no longer obstructs blood flow through ventricular vessels.

Conversely, right coronary arterial flow rate is highest during systole, because the aortic pressure driving flow increases more during systole (from 80 to 120 mmHg) compared to the right ventricular pressure, which opposes flow (from 0 to 25 mmHg).

O_2 extraction by the myocardium at rest is very high (65%) compared to other tissues (35%).

What factors determine coronary blood flow?

Pressure
> Coronary perfusion pressure; difference between aortic end-diastolic pressure and left ventricular end diastolic pressure
> Perfusion time; duration of diastole
> External compression.

Patency
> Vessel wall diameter
> Metabolic autoregulation related to vasoactive metabolites such as adenosine and nitric oxide

The amounts of metabolites are related to myocardial oxygen consumption

Neural input: α1-adrenergic receptors → vasoconstriction, and β2-adrenergic → vasodilatation

Drugs causing vasodilatation/vasoconstriction.

Flow

Blood viscosity.

How can coronary blood flow be measured?

1. *Clearance methods:* these are based on the Fick/Kety–Schmidt method and involve introducing an inert gas (usually nitrous oxide) into the circulation via the lungs and following the progressive saturation of cardiac tissue.
2. *Dilution methods:* thermodilution or dye dilution.
3. *Nuclear methods:* radionuclides such as xenon with coronary angiography. Thallium scan can indicate perfusion and technetium can indicate infarcted areas.
4. *Flowmeter techniques:* electromagnetic and Doppler flowmeters can be used.

10

Draw the oxygen dissociation curve.

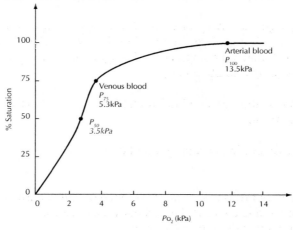

Diagram 10

> **Top tip**
> As always label the axis but in this case it is important to draw the curve shape accurately and mark the P_{50}, P_{75} and P_{100} points

What factors move it to the left and right?
The curve is shifted to the right by:

↑ H^+ ions, ↑ CO_2, ↑ temperature, ↑ 2,3-DPG

The curve is shifted to the left by:

↓ H^+ ions, ↓ CO_2, ↓ temperature, ↓ 2,3-DPG, Fetal Hb, Met Hb, CO Hb.

Why is the curve sigmoid in shape?
The purpose of an oxygen dissociation curve is to show the equilibrium of oxyhaemoglobin and non-bonded haemoglobin at various partial pressures.

There is cooperative binding between the oxygen and the four polypeptide subunits. The initial flat part of the curve occurs because the binding of the first oxygen molecule causes a small structural change to Hb facilitating the binding of subsequent oxygen molecules. As the maximum binding limit is approached, very little additional binding occurs and the curve levels out as the haemoglobin becomes saturated with oxygen. Hence the curve has a sigmoid shape.

What is the Bohr effect?
The Bohr effect describes the shift to the right of the oxyhaemoglobin curve associated with an increased PCO_2 and or a fall in pH. This favours oxygen delivery to the tissues.

What is the Haldane effect?
The Haldane effect describes the increased capacity of deoxyhaemoglobin to transport CO_2. This is due to the increased buffering ability of reduced Hb and the increased binding capacity of reduced Hb to CO_2.

What compensatory changes due to hypoxia occur at high altitude?
Immediate: hyperventilation leading to fall in PCO_2 and increase in alveolar PO_2 (by the alveolar gas equation).

Hours: renal elimination of bicarbonate and desensitisation of the chemoreceptors.

Later: polycythaemia, increased 2,3-DPG, increased capillary density particularly in muscle, increased mitochondrial density, increased pulmonary arterial pressures due to hypoxic pulmonary vasoconstriction, increased ventilatory capacity aided by the decreased density of air.

What effect do these compensatory changes have on the oxygen dissociation curve?

The hyperventilation results in a decreased CO_2 and therefore H^+ pushing the curve to the left. However, the increase in 2,3-DPG results in the curve being pushed to the right thereby allowing more oxygen to be delivered to the tissues.

Why is the oxyhaemoglobin curve relevant in pregnancy?

Fetal haemoglobin has a greater affinity for oxygen than adult haemoglobin, thus enhancing transfer of oxygen from the maternal circulation in the placenta. As a result the curve is left-shifted for fetal hemoglobin in comparison to the adult hemoglobin.

Pharmacology Answers

What is a local anaesthetic agent and how does it work?
A local anaesthetic is a drug which blocks the sodium channel thereby preventing nerve conduction. Unionised lipid-soluble drug passes through the phospholipid membrane and binds to sodium channels, thus preventing sodium entry during depolarisation, thereby stopping the propagation of the action potential.

How are local anaesthetics classified?
Local anaesthetics can be divided into esters and amides depending on the nature of the linkage between the aromatic lipophilic group and the hydrophilic group that local anaesthetics possess. Examples of esters are procaine, amethocaine and cocaine. Examples of amides are lignocaine and bupivacaine.

What are the recommended doses of lignocaine and bupivacaine?
The maximum recommended 'safe dose' of lignocaine is 3 mg/kg or 7 mg/kg if used with adrenaline.

The maximum recommended 'safe dose' of bupivacaine is 2 mg/kg.

Why does bupivacaine work more slowly than lignocaine?
The pKa or dissociation constant affects the onset time of local anaesthetic drugs.

The pKa value represents the pH at which the concentrations of the unionised base and the ionised base are equal. Bupivacaine has a pKa of 8.1 and therefore at lower pH values less drug will be unionised and therefore able to cross the phospholipid membrane resulting in a slower onset of block. Conversely, lignocaine has a pKa of 7.7 and therefore has a quicker onset of action.

What role does the racemic mixture play in the problem of bupivacaine toxicity?
Bupivacaine is much more cardiotoxic than other local anaesthetics. Ventricular arrhythmias and cardiac arrest are thought to be due to its effect on calcium and/or potassium channels (as well as sodium channels). Cardiac arrest due to bupivacaine toxicity may be very resistant to resus-

citation. Massive doses of adrenaline have been shown to be effective in animal studies in this situation. Bupivacaine has two isomers: R(+)-bupivacaine and S(–)-bupivacaine. The R(+) enantiomer is 3–4 times more likely to cause cardiotoxicity than S(–)-bupivacaine in rabbit hearts. Less cardiovascular disturbance has also been shown in humans with the S(–) form. Studies in sheep have shown a higher threshold for convulsions with the S(–) form. These safer features are not at the expense of efficacy.

In what way does inflammation affect local anaesthetic efficacy? Why?
The extracellular pH can alter the degree of ionisation and thus the lipid solubility of the drug. The local anaesthetic passes through the phospholipid membrane in an unionised form. The acidic environment created by inflammation and infection makes local anaesthetics more ionised and therefore less lipid soluble and less effective.

In addition, inflamed areas are more vascular and therefore any local anaesthetic used is more rapidly removed from the area.

What characteristics of local anaesthetics affect their onset of action, potency and duration of action?
pKa or dissociation constant: rapidity and onset

Lipid solubility: potency

Plasma and tissue binding: duration of action.

2

What are the uses of non-steroidal anti-inflammatory drugs?
Anti-inflammatory
Analgesia: Mild to moderate pain
                    Opioid-sparing effect
Antipyretic
Uricosuric.

How do NSAIDs work?
By inhibiting the enzyme cyclooxygenase (COX) thereby preventing the production of prostaglandins and thromboxanes from membrane phospholipids.

They are highly protein bound in the plasma and have low volumes of distribution.

Draw the pathway that they interrupt.

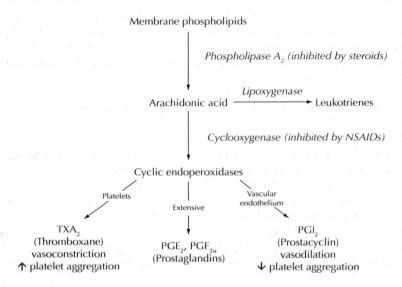

Membrane phospholipids

Phospholipase A$_2$ (inhibited by steroids)

Arachidonic acid ———*Lipoxygenase*———→ Leukotrienes

Cyclooxygenase (inhibited by NSAIDs)

Cyclic endoperoxidases

Platelets

Extensive

Vascular endothelium

TXA$_2$
(Thromboxane)
vasoconstriction
↑ platelet aggregation

PGE$_2$, PGF$_{2\alpha}$
(Prostaglandins)

PGI$_2$
(Prostacyclin)
vasodilation
↓ platelet aggregation

Diagram 11

What are the side-effects of NSAIDs? How can we avoid them?
Gastrointestinal intolerance: dyspepsia, gastric erosions, haematemesis, GI bleed

NSAID-sensitive asthma
Renal damage: urate retention, renal impairment, renal failure
Platelet function decreased and impaired coagulation and increased bleeding time
Hepatotoxicity
Skin reactions
Neurological symptoms
Drug interactions
Adverse drug reactions
Metabolic acidosis.

Side-effects can be avoided by judicious dosing, protective measures such as keeping the patient well hydrated, gastric protection agents and by using drugs with less harmful side-effects and more COX2 selectivity. There is a reduced risk of serious adverse GI effects with the COX2 inhibitors. (Some evidence suggests an increased risk of cardiovascular events.)

COX exists in two forms, COX1 and COX2. COX1 is the 'constitutive' form which is essential to normal bodily functions and is responsible for the production of prostaglandins, which are necessary for haemostasis, renal blood flow, gastric protection along with other roles (prostaglandins PGE_2 and PGI_2, and thromboxane TXA_2). COX2 is the 'inducible' form which is produced in response to tissue damage. It is the COX2 which has been targeted for the treatment of pain.

In which situations would you avoid giving patients NSAIDs?

Absolute contraindications
PET, hypovolemia, uncontrolled hypertension, NSAID-sensitive asthma, uncontrolled bleeding, renal compromise
Should be avoided
Elderly, diabetes, vascular disease and after cardiac, heptobiliary, renal or major vascular surgery (potential renal compromise).

Give some examples of selective NSAIDs
Celecoxib, rofecoxib

How does aspirin differ from other NSAIDs?
Aspirin is a derivative of salicylic acid, which is derived from willow bark.

It produces irreversible inhibition by acetylation of cyclooxygenase, the effects of which persist after the drug is cleared. Other NSAIDs cause reversible inhibition.

What are the features of an aspirin overdose? How can the overdose be treated?
CSF acidosis occurs, leading to hyperventilation and respiratory alkalosis with increased renal excretion of bicarbonate which also results in fluid and potassium loss, leading to dehydration and hypokalaemia.

Salicylism: confusion, dizziness, nausea, vomiting, tinnitus + deafness, sweating, tachycardia, hyperventilation.

(NB In children overdose of aspirin will depress the respiratory centre leading to respiratory acidosis and metabolic acidosis due to accumulation of lactic and pyruvic acid.)

Treatment of poisoning
100% oxygen, ABCD + Don't Forget the Glucose
Call for help
Contact poisons unit
Activated charcoal if presents within 1 h of ingestion
Gastric lavage up to 24 h after ingestion
Check salicylate levels
Bicarbonate
Urinary alkalisation with bicarbonate and monitor urine pH
(Avoid forced alkaline diuresis – can lead to pulmonary oedema)
Haemodialysis in severe cases.

Top tip
Check out the Medicine and Healthcare Regulatory agency website for up to date details on how to manage poisoning with other drugs.
http://www.mhra.gov.uk/

3

What factors affect the uptake of anaesthetic agents from inhaled gas into the blood?
Inhaled concentration
Alveolar minute volume
Diffusion
The blood/gas partition coefficient
The partial pressure of volatile in the pulmonary artery
The pulmonary blood flow
The V/Q match
The concentration effect
The second gas effect.

Draw a graph to indicate the relationship between the alveolar concentration and inspired concentration of a gas and the wash in times for different volatile agents.

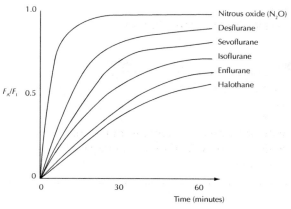

Diagram 12

What does the graph tell you about the solubility of the gas with the F_A/F_I closest to 1?
That the blood gas solubility is low and therefore equilibrium will be rapid. Rapid onset and rapid recovery.

Why is saturated vapour pressure (SVP) important? What is the SVP of desflurane?
The SVP indicates the degree of volatility. It is the pressure exerted by a vapour phase of a substance when in equilibrium with the liquid phase. SVP increases with temperature and therefore SVPs of volatile agents are quoted at standard temperature, usually 20°C. The SVP of desflurane is 88 kPa.

What does the oil gas coefficient indicate?
The potency of a gas. The higher the oil gas coefficient, the lower the MAC.

How is it relevant to how anaesthetics are believed to work?
Meyer–Overton theory states that inhalational anaesthetic agents act via the lipid-rich cells in the CNS and thus anaesthetic potency increases with lipid solubility.

Draw a graph of MAC versus oil gas coefficient and plot the main volatile agents.

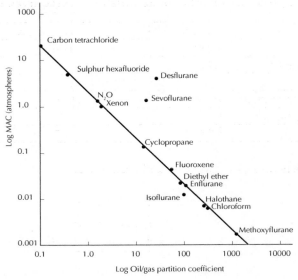

Diagram 13

What are the advantages and disadvantages of using desflurane?

Advantages

Desflurane has rapid onset and offset due to its low blood gas coefficient. Therefore, less volatile is needed once equilibrium is achieved and so in combination with low-flow anaesthesia for longer operations it can become economical since it is more expensive than other inhalational agents. Only 0.02% is metabolised.

Disadvantages

Desflurane may increase coronary blood flow (CBF) and intracranial pressure (ICP) although the response to CO_2 is preserved.

It can cause airway irritation and is therefore not recommended for induction of anaesthesia in children.

Pungent, unpleasant smell.

Along with the other volatile agents, it will cause a dose-dependent vasodilatation, hypotension, uterine relaxation and can precipitate malignant hyperthermia (MH).

It requires a special vaporiser due to its low boiling point.

Compare the physical properties of desflurane and sevoflurane.

	Sevoflurane	Desflurane
Mol. wt.	200	168
Boiling point (°C)	58	23
SVP (kPa)	21	88
Blood gas coefficient	0.69	0.42
Oil gas coefficient	53	19
MAC (%)	1.4–2.5	5–7

Draw the structure of sevoflurane and desflurane.

Desflurane

$$
\begin{array}{ccccc}
 & F & & H & F \\
 & | & & | & | \\
H - & C & - O - & C - & C - F \\
 & | & & | & | \\
 & F & & F & F \\
\end{array}
$$

Sevoflurane

$$
\begin{array}{ccc}
 & & F \\
 & & | \\
H & F - & C - F \\
| & & | \\
F - C - O - & C - H \\
| & & | \\
H & F - & C - F \\
 & & | \\
 & & F \\
\end{array}
$$

What are the problems associated with sevoflurane metabolism?

Sevoflurane interacts with soda lime to produce compounds A, B, C, D and E. Production is more likely at high temperature, high concentrations of sevoflurane, use of baralyme and low gas flows. Compound A has shown to be toxic in rats.

Less than 5% of sevoflurane is metabolised in the liver by cytochrome P450 but this metabolism leads to high levels of fluoride ions which it has been suggested could cause nephropathy. The enzyme P450 can be induced and therefore hasten metabolism.

> **Top tip**
> Write a list of the characteristics of the ideal volatile agent and then compare all of the commonly used agents with this list. It will help you remember their unique properties.

4

What is an inotrope?
A drug that affects myocardial contractility. There are positive and negative inotropes.

What is the difference between an inotrope and a vasopressor?
An inotrope affects contractility whereas a vasopressor affects systemic vascular resistance.

Classify inotropes.

Catecholamines
- Increase cAMP and intracellular calcium concentrations
- May be naturally occurring or synthetic
  - Adrenaline – α and β agonist
  - Noradrenaline – mainly α, some β agonist
  - Isoprenaline – β agonist only
  - Dopamine – α, β and D1 agonist
  - Dobutamine – mainly β1 agonist, weak α and β2 effect
  - Dopexamine – β2, D1 and D2 agonist.

Phosphodiesterase inhibitors
- Increase cAMP concentrations by preventing its breakdown
- Positive inotropism via PDE III and vasodilatation (inodilators)
- Little effect on myocardial oxygen demand

Specific – enoximone, amrinone, milrinone
Non-specific – aminophylline.

Cardiac glycosides
- Inhibit the action of the Na^+/K^+ATPase in cell membranes, increasing intracellular Na^+ which displaces bound intracellular calcium ions.

Calcium
- Has a transient positive inotropic effect by increasing intracellular calcium ions

Glucagon
- Causes increased cAMP concentrations and intracellular calcium release by acting on an unknown receptor.

Discuss dopexamine.

Dopexamine is used in the treatment of low cardiac output states and in acute heart failure. It is a synthetic dopamine analogue, presented as a clear solution of 10 mg/ml. Its main actions are arterial vasodilatation, positive inotropism and renal artery vasodilatation. It is an agonist at dopaminergic D1 and D2 receptors and therefore leads to relaxation of vascular smooth muscle in the renal, mesenteric, cerebral and coronary arterial beds (D1 effects) and stimulation of sympathetic D2 receptors, leading to decreased noradrenaline release. It also inhibits uptake of noradrenaline and has potent $\beta2$ adrenergic agonist activity.

System	Effect
Cardiovascular system	Positive inotrope and chronotrope, arterial vasodilatation, ↑ in coronary blood flow
Respiratory system	Bronchodilatation
Central nervous system	↑ Cerebral blood flow
Autonomic nervous system	↑ Splanchnic blood flow
Genitourinary system	↓ Renal vascular resistance leading to ↑ renal plasma flow

The dosage is 0.5–6 µg/kg per min and the $t_{1/2}$ = 5–10 min. The drug is extensively metabolised in the liver and excreted in bile and urine. The side-effects include: arrhythmias, angina, tremor, flushing, headache, nausea and vomiting.

Top tip

When presenting a drug follow a set pattern such as uses, presentation, concentration, main actions, mode of action, dose, routes of administration, effects on each system, side-effects, kinetics

---

In what situations do we give adrenaline?
As an inotrope
Anaphylaxis and bronchospasm
In cardiac arrest
With local anaesthetics
In croup/tracheitis.

What are the routes by which adrenaline can be given?
Intravenous, intramuscular, nebulised and endotracheal (endotracheal if no other route can be found, then at 3 times the normal dose given).

What effect does adrenaline have on systemic vascular resistance?
Adrenaline increases systemic vascular resistance.

What dose and concentration of adrenaline would you give for the treatment of anaphylaxis?
Adrenaline may be given intramuscularly in a dose of 0.5–1 mg (0.5–1 ml of 1:1000) and repeated every 10 min according to the arterial pressure and pulse until improvement occurs.

Alternatively, 50–100 µg intravenously (0.5–1 ml of 1:10,000) over 1 min has been recommended for hypotension with titration of further doses as required. Undiluted adrenaline 1:1000 should never be given intravenously.

What is the rationale for use of adrenaline in CPR
During CPR, adrenaline is given every 3–5 min – this reflects its half-life.

CPR produces only 10%–15% of normal cardiac output and during cardiac arrest there is also loss of vasomotor tone and venous pooling of blood. The highest priority in cardiac arrest is to maximise the available blood flow through the coronary arteries. The α-adrenergic activity of high-dose adrenaline produces peripheral vasoconstriction and thereby redistributes the available circulatory output centrally, increases coronary artery perfusion pressure and promotes coronary blood flow.

5

If I take this beaker of water, pretend it is a patient's blood and add my drug A to it, how do I calculate the volume of distribution of the drug?
The volume of distribution V_d is equal to the dose divided by the concentration at time zero C_0.

Let us assume a one-compartment model. What will happen to the concentration of the drug over time? Draw a graph to represent this. How can we make this graph easier to interpret?
The concentration of the drug will decline in an exponential fashion. This means that a constant proportion of the drug is removed per unit time.
The concentration is given by the following equation:

$C=C_0e^{-kt}$ (for a single-compartment model),
where C_0 is the concentration at time zero.
$t_{1/2}$ is the time required for the concentration of the drug to decline by 50%.
k is the slope of the graph and is the elimination rate constant, ie the fraction of drug present at any time that would be eliminated in unit time.

The reciprocal of k is the time constant τ, which is the time taken for C to fall to $1/e$ of its former value, if the initial rate of decline continued. $1/e$ is 37% of the former value.

The area under the curve (AUC) is equal to C_0 divided by the rate constant k.

Top tip
When drawing graphs:
1. Always start by drawing the axes
2. Then label the axes and put the units in brackets
3. Then mark the important points before drawing the curve or line

---

Pharmacokinetics

V_d = Volume of distribution

$$V_d = \frac{Xo}{Co} = \frac{\text{Amount of drug}}{\text{Concentration of drug}} = \frac{\text{dose}}{Co}$$

If we assume a one compartment model;

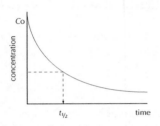

$t_{1/2}$ is the time at which the concentration is half what it was at time 0.

If we then take log entry of this graph, the graph becomes easier to interpret.

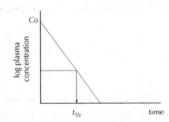

Diagram 14

How can we calculate the clearance?
Clearance is defined as the volume of plasma cleared per unit time

Clearance= $V_d \times k$

How can we calculate the half-life?
If $t_{1/2}=X_0/2=X_0e^{-kt_{1/2}}$, then divide by X_0 and take logs and you are left with $t_{1/2}=\ln2/k$.

ln2 is the natural logarithm.

What do you understand by the context sensitive half-life?
The time for the plasma concentration to decline by half after the termination of an infusion which has maintained a constant plasma concentration. Ultra short-acting drugs such as remifentanil are less affected by context (the infusion time).

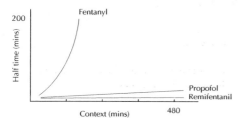

Diagram 15

What are the drawbacks of pharmacokinetic models?
They do not reflect physiological, ethnic and pathological variability.

There is no definite relationship between the plasma concentration and the pharmacological effect (pharmacodynamics).

What types of neuromuscular blocking drugs are there?
Neuromuscular blockers can be broadly divided into non-depolarising and depolarising agents. Non-depolarising agents can be divided into amino-steroids (examples rocuronium and vecuronium) and benzylisoquinolinium esters (examples atracurium and mivacurium).

How do their mechanisms of action differ?
Non-depolarising drugs are competitive antagonists at postsynaptic ACh receptors of the neuromuscular junction.

Depolarising drugs such as suxamethonium mimic the action of ACh at the ACh receptor but without rapid hydrolysis by acetylcholinesterase, instead waiting for hydrolysis by plasma cholinesterase. This depolarisation is what causes the classical fasciculation.

What can happen if you give a second dose of suxamethonium?
Dual or phase II block.

Features of non-depolarising blockade gradually replace those of depolarising blockade. The mechanism is unclear.

What are the advantages of rocuronium?
Rocuronium is an aminosteroid non-depolarising neuromuscular blocking drug. Its main advantage is its rapid onset (intubating conditions occur after an initial dose of 0.6 mg/kg in 100–120 seconds (blockade within 60 seconds at higher doses) with relaxation lasting 30–40 min. It has minimal cardiovascular effects and is mainly excreted unchanged in the bile.

What are the properties of an ideal neuromuscular blocker?
The ideal neuromuscular blocker:

Physical
    Stable at room temperature, in light
Pharmacological
    Non-depolarising action
    Rapid onset
    Short duration
    High potency
    Non-cumulative
    Minimal CVS side-effects
    No histamine release
    Spontaneous reversal
    Pharmacologically inactive metabolites
    Unaffected by renal or hepatic failure
    Safe in pregnancy
    Cheap and easy to produce.

7

What do we use benzodiazepines for in clinical practice?
Pre-medicant
Amnesia; anterograde
Part of a general anaesthetic
Sedation during minor procedures
Anticonvulsant
Anxiolysis/panic attacks
Hypnosis and insomnia.

What is the mechanism of action of benzodiazepines?
Benzodiazepines act by enhancing GABA-mediated inhibition of the brain and spinal cord especially of the limbic system.

GABA released from nerve terminals binds to $GABA_A$ receptors, the activation of which increases chloride ion transmission. The $GABA_A$ chloride complex also has a benzodiazepine receptor site. Occupation of this site by benzodiazepine agonists causes a conformational change in the GABA receptor enhancing the binding and the actions of GABA on the chloride conductance.

Why is temazepam preferred for night-time sedation compared with diazepam?
Temazepam has a half-life of 6 hours and so will cause less day-time somnolence compared with diazepam, which has a half-life of 24–48 hours.

Compare midazolam and diazepam.

	Midazolam	Diazepam
Uses	Induction, anxiety, premedication, sedation, anterograde amnesia	Induction, anxiety, premedication, sedation, status epilepticus
Presentation	Clear, colourless solution 2 or 5 mg/ml	Tablets of 2, 5, or 10 mg, as a syrup or as suppositories; IV diazepam is supplied as Diazemuls as an emulsion of the drug in soya bean oil
Dose	po 0.5 mg/kg im 0.08 mg/kg iv 0.1 mg/kg, titrated	po 2–60 mg/day in divided doses iv 10–30 mg
Onset	Fast, high lipid solubility Bioavailability, oral 44%	Medium, medium lipid solubility Bioavailability is 86%–100%
Half-life	1–3 hours	24–48 hours
Metabolism	To inactive compounds Rapid elimination	Active metabolites temazepam and nordiazepam

What kind of isomerism does midazolam display?
Midazolam is a structural isomer known as a tautomer – it is a dynamic isomer where two structural isomers exist in equilibrium.

How are benzodiazepines metabolised?
Benzodiazepines are metabolized in the liver by glucuronidation and oxidation. Metabolism often produces active metabolites especially with diazepam.

What are the principles of treating benzodiazepine poisoning?
Initial assessment
Monitor ABCD and secure airway if GCS <8
Consider whether co-poisons
Consider gastric lavage/charcoal
Contact poisons unit/ Seek ITU advice
Flumazenil is a specific benzodiazepine competitive antagonist. It can cause side-effects such as nausea, vomiting, dizziness, confusion, pulmonary oedema along with excessive excitement and convulsions. It has a short half-life so it can be used as an infusion if a long-acting benzodiazepine has been used.

What is an adverse drug reaction?
An adverse drug reaction (ADR) is an unwanted or harmful reaction experienced following the administration of a drug or combination of drugs and is suspected to be related to the drug. A serious ADR is defined as one that requires hospital admission, prolongs hospital stay, is permanently disabling, or results in death.

What is the term we use to describe a genetically determined adverse drug reactions?
Idiosyncrasy.

Give some examples of idiosyncratic drug reactions.
- Haemolysis with glucose 6-phosphatase dehydrogenase (G6PD) deficiency
- Prolongation of the action of suxamethonium with genetic variants
- Slow acetylators
- Malignant hyperthermia
- Acute hepatic porphyria.

Can you expand on the mechanism of idiosyncrasy in these examples

G6PD deficiency or favism
The absence or deficiency of this enzyme delays the regeneration of NADPH, which acts to protect the erythrocyte from the injurious effects of oxidative drugs.
Susceptible patients may develop haemolytic anaemia and jaundice.
Examples include sulphonamides, antimalarials, NSAIDs.

Suxamethonium apnoea
Ten possible genotypes for plasma cholinesterase, four alleles on chromosome 3:
- Normal Eu
- Atypical (dibucaine resistant) Ea
- Silent (Absent) Es
- Fluoride resistant Ef.

Slow acetylators
The hepatic enzyme N-acetyltransferase shows a genetic polymorphism. Can lead to toxic effects with isoniazid, hydralazine, phenelzine and certain sulphonamides.

Malignant hyperthermia
Rare but potentially fatal complication of anaesthesia. 1 in 200,000 in the UK. Autosomal dominant
Ryanodine receptor on chromosome 19
Trigger agents precipitate excessive Ca^{2+} release from sarcoplasmic reticulum.

Acute hepatic porphyria
Overproduction and excretion of porphyrins caused by enzyme defects in haem metabolic pathways.
Induces δ-aminolaevulinic synthetase → increased porphyrins.
Precipitants include barbiturates, phenytoin, alcohol and sulphonamides.

By what process would you manage and report a suspected adverse drug reaction?
The Committee on Safety of Medicines and Medicines and Healthcare products Regulatory Agency (MHRA) introduced the yellow card scheme which can be used to report any suspected drug reaction.
History and discussion with the patient plus advice/warning

Refer for genetic testing
Discuss with senior anaesthetist
Anaesthetic follow-up.

What does this symbol mean when next to a drug in the *British National Formulary*?

The black triangle indicates new drugs which are being intensively monitored in order to confirm the risk/benefit profile of the drug.

Name some drugs that are known to cause emesis.
Nitrous oxide
Etomidate
Neostigmine
Morphine and opioids
Cytotoxic drugs.

Explain the various neural inputs that result in vomiting.

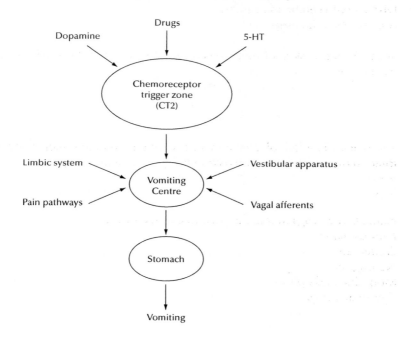

Diagram 16: Neural inputs that result in vomiting

Neurotransmitters involved in nausea and vomiting can be thought of as central or peripheral. Centrally (inside the blood–brain barrier) is the vomiting centre, which has muscarinic acetylcholine receptors and histamine receptors. The chemoreceptor trigger zone (which lies outside the blood–brain barrier) has dopamine (D2) and 5-HT$_3$ receptors. Peripherally in the stomach there are dopamine and 5-HT3 receptors.

What neurotransmitters are involved in nausea and vomiting?
Dopamine
5HT
Acetylcholine.

What anti-emetics do you know of? What is their mode of action?
Anti-emetics can be classified by their site of action.
Dopamine antagonists: metoclopramide, prochlorperazine, droperidol, domperidone.
Antihistamines: promethazine, cyclizine.
Anticholinergics: hyoscine.
5-HT$_3$ antagonists: ondansetron, granisetron (?metoclopramide in high doses).
Corticosteroids: dexamethasone.
Cannabinoids: nabilone.

How can we administer anti-emetics?
Anti-emetics can be given orally, intravenously, intramuscularly, rectally or transdermally.

Name any drugs that can be administered transdermally.
Fentanyl, glyceryl trinitrate, amethocaine (Ametop), prilocaine, nicotine and lignocaine (EMLA), hormone replacement therapy.

What is a dose–response curve?
A dose–response curve can be used to explain the relationship between the dose of a drug and the resultant response. A logarithmic scale is usually used for the x axis and the position on the x axis is related to the potency of a drug; the maximal height is related to the efficacy and the slope is related to the receptor activation required for drug effect.

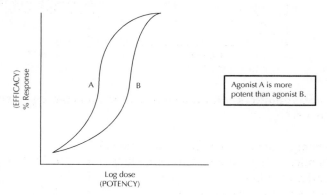

Diagram 17: Agonist A and B

Draw a curve to indicate a competitive reversible antagonist and one to indicate a competitive irreversible antagonist? Give examples of such drugs.

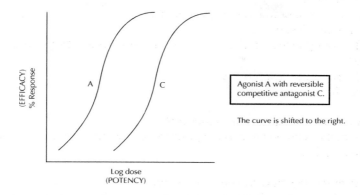

Diagram 18: Agonist A with antagonist C reversible eg atropine, atracurium, atenolol

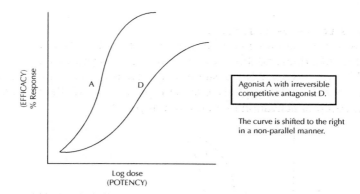

Diagram 19: Agonist A with antagonist D irreversible eg phenoxyben-zamine on α receptors

Give an example of non-competitive antagonism.
Direct chemical combination such as metallic ions and chelating agents, heparin and protamine
Via receptor systems, eg gallamine.

What are partial agonists? Draw a curve to indicate the response. Give an example.

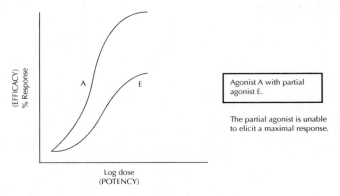

Diagram 20: Partial agonist E, eg buprenorphine.

What is an inverse agonist? Draw a graph to indicate the response.

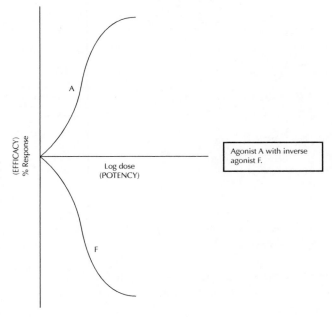

Diagram 21: Inverse agonist F.

An inverse agonist has receptor affinity but negative intrinsic activity and therefore produces pharmacological effects opposite to those of a full agonist, eg flumazenil.

Physics and Clinical Measurement Answers

What do you understand by the Venturi effect?
The Venturi principle describes entrainment of fluid through a side arm into an area of low pressure caused by constriction in a tube.

What is the Bernoulli principle?
At a constriction in a tube the flow will increase and the kinetic energy will rise. Since energy is conserved or remains the same at this constriction, the potential energy will fall and therefore the pressure will also fall. It is this fall in pressure which causes the Venturi effect by entraining flow.

How does a Venturi mask use these principles to deliver different oxygen concentrations?
Venturi masks are also known as 'fixed performance devices' as they can deliver a predetermined and fixed oxygen concentration to the patient. The size of the constriction or aperture in the mask will affect the amount of air entrained and therefore the final oxygen concentration. The devices are colour coded to indicate the percentage of oxygen delivered at a particular fresh gas flow: green 60% to blue 24%.

What is the entrainment ratio?
The entrainment ratio is defined by the ratio of entrained flow to driving flow.

What is the usual entrainment ratio in Venturi masks?
(O_2 flow from the wall)/(Entrained air flow) = $(F_iO_2-0.2)/(1-F_iO_2)$

For example, if the oxygen flow is 10 l/min and $F_iO_2=0.6$, the ratio will be 1:1; ie for each litre of oxygen, 1 litre of air will be entrained.

What are the other uses of Venturi?
The Venturi principle is used in Venturi oxygen masks, suction equipment, scavenging equipment, nebulisers, ventilators, ejector flowmeters and vacuum cleaners.

If Venturi masks are fixed performance devices, give an example of a variable performance device. What factors will affect the final F_iO_2 in a variable performance device?
An example of a variable performance device is a Hudson mask.

Factors affecting final F_iO_2 are:
1. Oxygen supply flow rate.
2. Pattern of ventilation. Pause between expiration and inspiration allows mask to fill with oxygen.
3. Patient's inspiratory flow. Oxygen is diluted by air drawn in through the holes when inspiratory flow rate exceeds flow of oxygen supply.
4. How tight the mask fits on the face.

What is the Coanda effect?
The Coanda effect, also known as 'boundary layer attachment', is the tendency of a stream of fluid to stay attached to a convex surface, rather than follow a straight line in its original direction. Discovered in 1930 by Henri Coanda, a Romanian aircraft engineer, the phenomenon has many practical applications in fluidics and aerodynamics. It can also be used to explain the distribution of air in the pulmonary tree after a constriction in the bronchiole, as the flow will stream along one fork of the division, leading to unequal distribution of gas flow.

Define humidity.
Absolute humidity is the amount of water vapour per unit volume of gas at a given temperature and pressure in g/m^3 or mg/l.

Relative humidity (%) is the absolute humidity divided by the amount present when the gas is fully saturated at the same temperature and pressure.

What are the normal values for humidity in the upper trachea and the alveoli?
Upper trachea 34 g/m^3, alveoli 43 g/m^3.

How can we measure humidity? Describe how each method works.
Humidity can be measured using a hygrometer.

The types of hygrometer are:
- Relative humidity

  Hair hygrometer: Uses the effect of humidity on hair expansion and contraction to measure humidity.

  Wet and dry bulb hygrometer: Uses the difference in temperature between a thermometer with a wet bulb and one with a dry bulb to measure humidity. As water evaporates from the wet bulb, the bulb cools producing a temperature difference between the thermometers. The amount of evaporation depends on the relative humidity of the air.

  Humidity transducers: Electrical resistance or capacitance of a membrane changes with humidity.

  Mass spectroscopy

- Absolute humidity

  Regnault's hygrometer: The air under test is bubbled through ether in a silver tube. This has a cooling effect leading to condensation. The temperature at which condensation occurs is known as the 'dew point.' The dew point represents the temperature at which ambient air is fully saturated. Relative humidity and absolute humidity can then be deduced.

Top tip
You can draw pictures to illustrate your answers.

What is the humidity achievable by HMEF?
About 25 g/m^3.

What is the normal operating theatre humidity? What are the risks in theatre if the humidity too low?
The normal relative humidity in the operating theatre is 50%–60%. There is increased risk of sparks and electrical fires if humidity is too low.

3

What methods are used to measure volatile gases? Which is the most common in a modern anaesthetic machine? Describe how each method works.
There are a number of ways to measure volatile gases; infrared analysis is the most common.

Infrared analysis

A gas will absorb infrared radiation causing it to vibrate if it consists of more than one atom. Each molecule has a unique fingerprint pattern of infrared absorption that follows the Beer–Lambert law. It can be used to measure CO_2 as well as volatile agents.

Mass spectrometry

Sample gas passing through an ionising chamber is bombarded by an electron beam. Charged molecules pass through a strong magnetic field. The amount of deflection is proportional to mass.

Raman spectrometry

The Raman effect. When light interacts with the gas molecule its change is rotational and vibrational energy is characteristic.

Photoacoustic spectroscopy

This exposes a gas to three beams of radiation, which are absorbed leading to audio signals.

Piezoelectric effect

The change in resonant frequency of a crystal of quartz in the presence of anaesthetic agents is proportional to the amount of volatile present.

Refractometers

A light beam is split and passed through two chambers.

How do we measure oxygen?

Spectrophotometric, eg pulse oximeter; oxygen content: Van Slyke apparatus.
Clark/Polarographic electrode
Fuel cell
Paramagnetic analyser.

Tell me how the Clark electrode works.

CLARK / POLAROGRAPHIC ELECTRODE
At constant temp 37°C.

0.6V

Flow of electric
current α O_2 partial pressure

Ag/Ag | Cl
anode

Ag + Cl⁻
⟶ AgCl + e⁻

⊖

KCI

Platinum cathode – emits electrons
$O_2 + 2H_2O + 4e^- = 4OH^-$
(with plastic membrane to avoid
protein deposits)

KCl + OH = KOH + Cl⁻

Diagram 22: The flow of electrical current is proportional to the oxygen partial pressure.

Top tip
Be ready to talk about any method of measurement you mention.

4

What is ultrasound?
Transmission and reflection of high-frequency longitudinal mechanical waves in tissues to give images due to reflection from the surfaces between different tissues.

What is the Doppler effect/shift?
The Doppler effect is the increase in observed frequency of a signal when the signal source approaches the observer and the decrease as the source moves away.

Why is the Doppler effect relevant to us?

The Doppler effect can be used with ultrasound to determine velocities and flow rates of moving substances. The probe has an emitter and detector at the probe tip.

$V = \delta f \, v / 2f \cos \theta$.

Give some examples of how the Doppler is used clinically.

Oesophageal Doppler is used to measure cardiac output and guide fluid management in major surgery and in ITU.
Transcranial Doppler to measure coronary blood flow.
Echocardiography Doppler – uses colour Doppler to give information about the direction as well as the velocity of flow.
Arterial flow – is used to evaluate flow through arteries and can give a measure of systolic and diastolic pressure.
Imaging – in the duplex Doppler form it can also provide a picture of the blood vessel and surrounding organs.

Power Doppler is another newer mode combining colour and duplex Doppler; it is used to evaluate blood flow through vessels within solid organs.

What is a pulse oximeter?

It is a device used to determine oxygen saturation during oximetry and gives a plethysmographic pulse waveform.

How does it work?

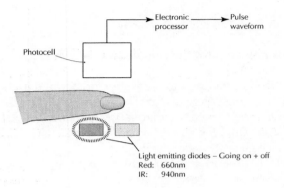

Viva Physics – Oximeter

Diagram 23: The Beer–Lambert laws.

Beer's law: Absorption of a given thickness of a solution of a given concentration is the same as twice the thickness of half the concentration.
Lambert's law: Each layer of equal thickness absorbs an equal fraction of radiation which passes through it.

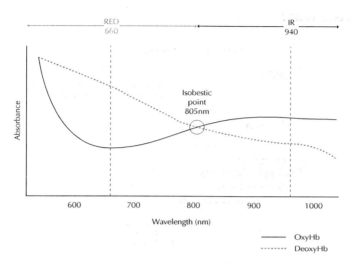

Diagram 24: Oxygenated (oxyHb) and deoxygenated haemoglobin (deoxyHb) have different absorbance spectra. Comparison of absorbance at different wavelengths allows estimation of the relative concentrations of oxyHb and deoxyHb. In infrared light (940 nm), the absorbance of oxyHb is greater than that of deoxyHb. The points where the absorbances for the two forms of Hb are identical, known as the 'isosbestic point', are 590 and 805 nm.

How does the pulse oximeter compensate for ambient light?
The light-emitting diodes (LEDS) go on and off in rapid sequence with a pause at high frequency. The pause allows the photocell and electronic processor to compensate for ambient light.

What can lead to inaccuracies in the pulse oximeter reading?
Patient factors
Environment factors
> Movement (eg shivering), electrical interference (eg diathermy), external light, venous congestion, ↓ pulsatile flow (vasoconstriction or peripheral vascular disease), nail varnish or false nails, skin staining/colouring (eg Henna Black>Red), a very low S_pO_2<50%.

Non-functioning Hb: carboxyhaemoglobin and methaemoglobin.
CarboxyHb → S_pO_2 falsely high.
Methaemoglobin and bilirubin: counted as HbO, → S_pO_2 falsely low.

S_pO_2 is not affected by jaundice, dark skin, or anaemia.

What are the risks with pulse oximeter use?
Thermal: overheating of the LED or current leakage can lead to burns.
Topical: due to product material or chemicals for cleaning.
Mechanical: due to pressure exerted by the probe.
Infective: cross-contamination between patients if not adequately cleaned.
Anatomical: thumb/finger dislocations if probe pulled off, toe deformity (in children).

What monitors do you consider essential to the safe conduct of anaesthesia?
I would follow the Association of Anaesthetists of Great Britain and Ireland (AAGBI) guideline for recommendations for standards of monitoring during anaesthesia. The monitoring standards are:

Observation by anaesthetist: mucosal colour, pupil size, response to surgical stimulus, chest wall movement, reservoir bag movement, palpation of pulse, auscultation of breath sounds and where appropriate measurement of urinary output (UO) and blood loss.

Pulse oximeter
NIBP (non-invasive blood pressure)
ECG (electrocardiograph)
ETCO$_2$ (capnograph)

Gas analysis
The following must also be available:

A nerve stimulator whenever a muscle relaxant is used.
A means of measuring the patient's temperature.

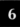

What do you understand by the term flow?
Flow is the amount of fluid moving per unit time. Flow can be laminar or turbulent.

What is the difference between laminar and turbulent flow?

Laminar flow
- Smooth orderly flow in a straight line in one direction without eddy currents
- Fluid flows parallel to the vessel wall
- Velocity is highest in the centre of the vessel, decreasing towards the periphery and approaching zero at the wall (parabolic velocity profile)
- The type of flow seen in smooth tubes at low flows
- Affected by viscosity.

Turbulent flow
- Flow is less organised, with eddy currents causing fluid flow in all directions although there is a general progression along the tube
- Occurs at high flow rates (where the critical velocity is exceeded), sharp angles, branching points and where there are changes in diameter or irregularities in the tube
- Affected by changes in density
- Compared with laminar flow, a greater pressure difference is required to maintain the same flow rate (ie there is a greater resistance to flow).

What equations do you know that explain the different types of flow?
Laminar flow through a tube is described by the Hagen–Poiseuille equation: $V = \Delta P \pi r^4 / 8 \eta l$, where V = rate of flow, ΔP = pressure gradient along tube, r = radius of tube, η = viscosity of fluid and l = length of tube.

For turbulent flow: flow rate is proportional to $\Delta P(r^2)/\Delta \rho$ where ΔP = pressure gradient along tube, r = radius of tube and ρ = density of fluid.

What is the Reynolds' number?
Reynolds' number = vpd/η where v = linear velocity, p = gas density, d = diameter of tube and η = gas viscosity. Reynolds' number is used to predict whether flow is laminar or turbulent. If it is greater than 2000, turbulent flow is likely. A value less than 1000 is associated with laminar flow. Between 1000 and 2000 both types of flow occur.

What is the critical velocity?
The critical velocity is the flow above which laminar flow in a tube becomes turbulent. At critical velocity, the Reynolds' number is >2000.

What devices do we use to measure flow? How can we classify them?

Type of flowmeter	Examples
Constant orifice, variable pressure	Simple pressure gauge Pneumotachograph Pitot tubes
Constant pressure, variable orifice	Rotameter Heidbrink flowmeter Peak flow meter
Variable pressure, variable orifice	Watersight flowmeter
Constant pressure, constant orifice	Bubble flowmeter
Other	Thermistor flowmeter Ultrasonic flowmeter

What is a rotameter?
A rotameter is a constant-pressure, variable-orifice device used to measure gas flow in the anaesthetic machine accurately. It consists of a tapered glass tube containing a bobbin or a ball.

Where do you read the gas flow from when you have a bobbin or a ball?
The top of a bobbin and the middle of a ball.

In which positions will a rotameter function?
Only in the upright position.

What safety features are employed in flowmeters?

Control knobs
Are labelled and colour coded.

Oxygen knob is larger, protrudes and has a different shape, often ridged (so it can be found in the dark!).

Oxygen knob is always on the left-hand side of the block in the UK.

The torque needed to operate the control knobs meets a UK safety standard so that it is high enough to try to avoid accidental re-adjustment.

Gas
Oxygen-nitrous oxide interlinking system – makes it impossible to deliver a hypoxic mixture.

Oxygen is the last gas to be delivered to the mixed gas flow, so that if there is a gas leak the chance of a hypoxic mixture being delivered to the patient is minimised.
Calibrated for each gas for highest accuracy.

Components/design

Flow restrictors are fitted downstream of the flowmeter to prevent back pressure being exerted on the flowmeter and producing inaccurate readings.

Anti-static materials and a filter to remove dirt are present in order to prevent the bobbin or ball sticking to the wall of the flowmeter causing inaccurate readings.

There should be good exposure of the top of the glass tubes to avoid concealment of bobbins so that high flow rates of gases are not hidden.

7

Here are photos of measuring devices *(see question 7 page 259)*. What do they measure? Name each type of instrument and describe how it works.
You are shown photographs of:
    A. tympanic thermometer
    B. mercury thermometer
    C. nasopharyngeal probe.

A mercury thermometer relies on the principle that the volume of mercury will change in proportion to the temperature change. It is effective in the range $-39°C$ to about $250°C$.

A nasopharyngeal probe has a thermistor at its tip, which is a semiconductor device that has a reducing resistance with increasing temperature, ie a negative temperature coefficient.

A tympanic thermometer relies on the principle that the amount of radiation emitted is proportional to temperature.

How can we classify the ways in which temperature is measured?
Ways of measuring temperature can be divided into electrical or non-electrical.

Electrical means are:
1. Platinum resistance thermometer
2. Thermistor
3. Thermocouple.

Non-electrical means are:

Liquid expansion
      Mercury thermometer
      Alcohol thermometer
      Gas thermometer

Dial thermometers
      Bimetallic strip, eg thermostat
      Based on Bourdon gauge

Chemical
      Liquid crystal

Other
      Infrared thermometry.

How does a thermocouple work?
A thermocouple relies on the 'Seebeck effect', which states that the production of voltage between two dissimilar conductors is proportional to the temperature. The circuit consists of a measuring thermocouple junction and reference electrode. It is usually made from copper and constantan.

Where can temperature be measured?
Skin
Axilla
Temporal artery thermometry
Tympanic membrane
Nasopharynx
Oropharynx
Oesophagus
Blood
Bladder
Rectum.

Where can you get an accurate core temperature reading?
Core temperature can be measured from the rectum, oesophagus, tympanic membrane or the bladder.

What are the temperature scales that you know of? Tell me about them.

Fahrenheit
According to this scale ice melts at 32°F, body temperature is 100°F and water boils at 212°F.

Celsius or centigrade
0°C is the melting point of ice and 100°C is the boiling point of water.

Kelvin: the absolute temperature scale
The unit 'kelvin' is defined as 1/273.16 of the triple point of water. The scale is defined by two points: absolute zero and the triple point of water. Absolute zero is defined as being precisely 0 K and –273.15 °C. The triple point is the temperature and pressure at which three phases (gas, liquid and solid) may coexist in thermodynamic equilibrium which is 273.16 K at 611.2 Pa (0.01°C).

8

What types of breathing system do you know of?
Breathing systems can be classified into open, semiopen, semiclosed or closed. Mapleson classified semiclosed breathing systems into A–E.

Draw the outline of a circle breathing system.
The key parts are an absorber, unidirectional valves and an exhaust valve.

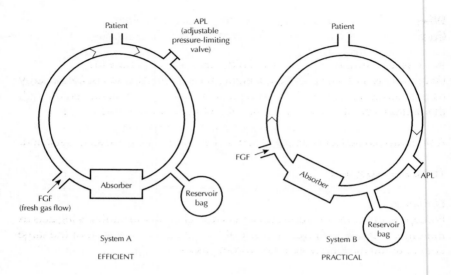

System A EFFICIENT — System B PRACTICAL

Diagram 25

System A is more efficient, system B is less efficient but more practical as the APL valve is further away from the patient and therefore dead space and alveolar gases mix before reaching it.

What is low-flow anaesthesia?
Low-flow anaesthesia is defined as ≤3 l/min fresh gas flow. Minimal flow is 0.5 l/min as basal requirements are 250 ml/min.

What are the advantages and disadvantages of low-flow anaesthesia?

Advantages
Economical: gases and volatiles
Detection: early detection of leaks in the system with IPPV
Humidity and warmth are retained
Ecological: decreased pollution
Easy to use now there is routine ET and inspired gas monitoring.

Disadvantages
Accumulation of substances
> Methane, acetone, hydrogen, alcohol, carbon monoxide, compound A and solvent from orthopaedic cement can build up.

Slow changes in anaesthetic concentrations.
Must give sufficiently high flow to denitrogenate at start of anaesthesia.

330

9

What is diathermy? What types of diathermy do you know of?

Diathermy is a device used to coagulate blood vessels, and cut and destroy tissues during surgery by the heating of an electrical current passed through them. It uses an alternating current with a frequency of 0.5–1 MHz.

A sine wave is used for cutting and damped or pulsed sine wave for coagulation.

There are two types:

Unipolar

Forceps act as one electrode and a plate attached to the patient's leg acts as the other electrode. Current density at this site is low because of the large area of tissue through which the current passes.

Bipolar

Current is passed across tissue held between the two tips of one pair of forceps.

When is unipolar diathermy used and when is bipolar diathermy used?

Bipolar is used for more delicate surgery, eg eye surgery or neurosurgery. Bipolar is usually incapable of cutting since it uses a lower power.

Unipolar diathermy can inhibit pacemaker function so in patients with pacemakers bipolar is usually used. If unipolar must be used the plate should be placed as far from the heart as possible to ensure current flow is not across the chest.

Why does diathermy not affect the cardiac and skeletal muscle?

The current density is kept high at the site of intended damage by using small electrodes, eg forceps tips.

You are shown two plates (one for a child, one for an adult). Where should the plate be placed and why? Discuss the current density.

The plate should be placed over a vascular, muscular area. Muscle is a better conductor of electricity than adipose tissue. Adequate tissue perfusion promotes electrical conductivity and dissipates heat. It should be as close to the operative site as possible and on the same side of the patient as the operative site.

If the plate area is reduced then the current density is increased and there is a higher risk of burns.

Ohm's law states that voltage = current × resistance ($V=IR$).
The heat energy produced = (current)2 × resistance ($E=I2R$).

What is a capacitor?
A capacitor is composed of conductors separated by an insulator. It may be charged by a potential difference but will not allow direct current to flow until it is discharged. It is used in defibrillators and in some diathermy machines.

Why is there a capacitor in the diathermy circuit?
A capacitor acts as a safety feature to prevent mains current flowing through the circuit and increasing the risk of burns. The patient circuit is isolated. It acts as a short circuit at diathermy frequencies (300 kHz to 3 MHz) but acts as an open circuit at mains frequencies (50 Hz). There is still a risk of burns if the patient touches a metal, because of capacitive coupling.

What are the hazards associated with diathermy?
Interference with monitoring and pacemakers
Burns
    If plate incorrectly attached
     Accidental activation of diathermy
Ignition of flammable substances.

Name the following electrical symbols.

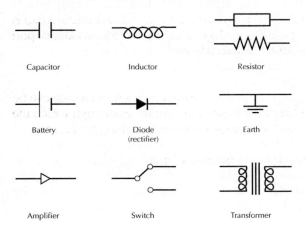

Capacitor	Inductor	Resistor
Battery	Diode (rectifier)	Earth
Amplifier	Switch	Transformer

10

How do we measure CO_2?
There are direct and indirect methods.

Direct: Severinghaus CO_2 electrode
Indirect: Mass spectrometry, infrared analyser (capnograph), interferometer, chromatography, Siggaard–Andersen nomogram, Van Slyke apparatus.

Tell me how the infrared analyser works.
The amount of infrared light absorbed by the sample gas is proportional to the amount of gas present and is determined by comparing the emergent beams by a photodetector from the sample and reference chamber.

The peak absorption wavelength of CO_2 is 4.28 µm.

What is collision broadening and how do we prevent it causing reading errors?
The CO_2 molecules absorb their rotational and vibrational energy as they absorb infrared. If the gases contain nitrous oxide, it is possible for energy to be transferred to the nitrous oxide when the molecules collide. This results in the CO_2 molecules absorbing more energy than if nitrous oxide was not present. Most analysers provide compensation for this effect.

What types of capnograph are there?

Side stream
Draws a sample at 150 ml/min via a tube to the analyser. A moisture trap is present to prevent inaccuracies caused by water and there is an exhaust port to return the gases to the patient after analysis.

Main stream
A special connector is incorporated into the breathing system which can be bulky. It incorporates a channel with sapphire windows through which the infrared beam passes directly into the gases in the breathing attachment.

What do the following capnograph traces indicate?
1. Normal
2. Malignant hyperpyrexia
3. Raised baseline, CO_2 rebreathing.

Clinical Answers

A 60-year-old woman with asthma for emergency repair of detached retina. How would you assess an asthmatic preoperatively?

History:
>   Hospital and ITU admissions with asthma and frequency of these admissions
>   Drug history (DHx)
>   Level of asthma control – previous and current
>   Triggering factors
>   Exercise tolerance
>   Recent viral respiratory tract infection (RTI) – postpone if still symptomatic
>   Compliance with Rx
>   Recent course of steroids
>   Allergies and other atopy
>   Smoking
>   NSAID effect on asthma

Examination
>   PEFR
>> Variability in PEFR should be assessed
>> >20% suggests poor control

Investigationsw
>   CXR
>   PEFR and reversibility; compare with predicted values for age, sex and height
>   ABG

Anaesthetics technique
>   Avoid histamine-releasing agents such as atracurium, morphine
>   Consider local in severe asthma and avoid GA
>   If GA, ETT vs LMA depending on severity of asthma
>   Elective surgery should only take place if the asthma is well controlled.

Wanted – lots of detail about PEFR measurement.

How would you treat a severe asthmatic?
β-agonists: short-acting salbutamol, longer-acting salmeterol
Steroids: inhaled beclomethasone, oral steroids
Anticholinergics: ipratropium bromide (Atrovent)
Aminophylline
Leukotriene drugs
Disodium cromoglicate
Magnesium
Ketamine
Volatile agents
Heliox.

What are the side-effects of salbutamol if used in high doses?
Tachycardia, tremor, anxiety and hypokalemia

Which is more important to continue, the β-agonist or steroids?
The steroid is more important to continue as it needs to be given regularly to be effective.

If patients are on inhalers then they can be converted to nebulisers in the perioperative period.

Is a CXR an important investigation in this scenario?
Yes as there is a risk of pneumothorax.

Top tip
Check out specialist society website for guidelines of treatment of diseases
The British Thoracic Society has up to date information
http://www.brit-thoracic.org.uk

How would you anaesthetise this patient?
Consider RA vs GA.

Consider ETT vs LMA. Since the tracheal tube itself may cause bronchospasm many advocate, if possible, avoiding intubation altogether. This will depend on the type of surgery and the severity of asthma.

Ensure adequate depth of anaesthesia at induction and at the start of the surgical stimulus to avoid bronchospasm.

A number of induction agents are safe in asthma: propofol and ketamine cause bronchodilatation. Thiopentone should be avoided as it has been implicated in worsening bronchospasm.

Muscle relaxant

Maintenance: inhalational gases are bronchodilators

Avoid β-blockers.

What is your postoperative care for a severe asthmatic?
HDU/ITU

Are they safely extubatable? Full examination prior to extubation.

Is there adequate analgesia or a regional block?

Reinstitute normal medications in nebuliser or IV form if necessary.

Physiotherapy.

Critical incident: there is a sudden increase in airway pressures. What is your approach to this situation?
Call for help, 100% oxygen.

Start at patient end: examine patient checking for air entry both sides and listen for bronchospasm and whether the ET tube is down the right main bronchus; check breathing system for kinks or blockages; transfer to alternative breathing system if necessary.

When you auscultate the chest you discover there is severe bronchospasm.
What action will you take?
Methods of bronchodilatation

    Anaesthetic drugs (deepen with volatile)

    β-agonists

    Aminophylline

    Magnesium.

On further auscultation you discover that there is hyper-resonance and absent breath sounds on the right-hand side of the chest. What is your diagnosis and what will you do?
This is a life-threatening emergency as I suspect a tension pneumothorax.

Management of tension pneumothorax
Large-bore cannula /or needle inserted at the 2nd intercostal space in the midaxillary line.

Expect to hear whoosh of air as the needle is removed.

100% oxygen, ABC.

> **Top tip**
> Convey to the examiner that you understand the gravity of the situation by stating that THIS IS A LIFE-THREATENING EMERGENCY!

What are the causes of a pneumothorax in the perioperative period that could be caused by the anaesthetist?
Intrapulmonary rupture
>High airway pressures during IPPV

Injury to the visceral pleura
>Fractured ribs
>Regional anaesthesia
>CVP insertion
>Tracheostomy.

2

Do you give blood to your patients? Do you discuss this with them preoperatively?
Yes I do but I would not give blood to a patient unless I felt it was absolutely necessary since blood transfusion carries significant risks.

In my preoperative visit I would check whether the patient has any objection to blood transfusion or has had any reaction to previous blood transfusion. I would check whether they carry an antibody card or know of any abnormal antibodies they carry.

The transfusion trigger will depend on the patient. In those with cardiovascular disease I would aim for a trigger of 8 g/dl and in other patients the trigger would be 7 g/dl but this would be influenced by local policy.

What happens when you ask for the blood to be group and saved?
Blood is sent to the blood bank, with minimum hand-labelled patient identification including correctly spelt names, DOB, hospital number, and is signed by the person who took the blood. The testing is called group and screen because the blood is tested for ABO and D groups, an antibody screen (indirect or in vitro Coombs' test) and a comparison is made with these results and any historical record. The is kept for 5–7 days and longer in some situations.

Tell me about the ABO blood group system.
Blood is grouped by antigens A, B, AB or O. Group O has no antigens and used to be called the universal donor (this does not account for the other antigens present and so is a dated term). Patients with group O can only receive blood group O themselves. Blood group AB has A and B antigens but does not make any ABO antibodies and so these patients do not discriminate against any other ABO type and are therefore the universal recipient. Groups O and A are the most common in the UK and there are genetic variations.

An **antigen** is any substance capable of inducing a specific immune response. It is found on the surface of the red cell.
An **antibody** is an immunoglobulin which is involved in immuno-logical defence. ABO antibodies are predominantly IgM and are found in the plasma.

What happens when you ask for blood to be cross matched?
Cross matching involves the selection of suitable units for compatibility testing. This involves mixing a sample of the recipient's blood with a sample of the donor's blood and checking to see if the mixture agglutinates, or forms clumps. There are currently 29 blood group systems (including the ABO and Rh systems). Thus, in addition to the ABO antigens and Rhesus antigens, many other antigens are expressed on the red blood cell surface membrane.

What types of blood are available to you when you need to give a blood transfusion?
O Rhesus negative Reserved for life-threatening emergencies especially in obstetrics because of the later risk of haemolytic disease of the newborn.
O Rhesus positive Life-threatening emergencies if known to be RhD-positive from previous records.
Group specific Rapidly issued uncrossmatched blood. Emergency ABO and D typing may not prevent minor incompatibilities.
Type specific Own blood or full cross match.

Here is an empty blood bag. Go through what you would do to check the blood.
Check patient's wrist band, consent and notes.
Check the details are the same.

Ask second trained person to check with me and use the compatibility form.

Check the Hospital number, name, DOB, blood group, expiry date, pack number.

Check the blood for signs of discoloration or bag interference.

The check is of extreme importance since incompatibility carries a significant morbidity and mortality.

How is blood stored?

Blood is stored in plastic collection bags permeable to CO_2. It is stored at 2–6°C. The survival time of the red cells is dependent on the storage solution.

One of the older methods of storage is citrate phosphate and dextrose (CPD). Later adenine was added creating CAPD, which increases cell ATP thereby increasing red cell survival to 35 days.

These days most blood is stored as SAGM – saline, adenine, glucose and mannitol. Used to resuspend concentrated red cells after removal of plasma (to be removed for other blood products) from CPD-anticoagulated blood. Saline suspends the red cells, glucose provides a substrate for metabolism and mannitol prevents haemolysis. Red cell survival is 35 days.

What is autologous blood transfusion?

Autologous means related to self. Autologous blood transfusion is the use of cell salvage or predonation of blood.

Why is blood leucodepleted?

Since 1999 all blood components have been leucodepleted in an attempt to decrease the potential risk of transfusion-transmitted variant Creutzfeldt-Jakob disease (vCJD).

What is the definition of a massive blood transfusion?

This is defined as the acute administration of more than 1.5 times the patient's blood volume, or replacement of the patient's total blood volume within 24 hours.

What is your management of a massive blood loss?
See Appendix 2 Blood transfusion and the anaesthetist AAGBI 2005

Call for help: on site
Restore circulating volume: large-bore cannula, insert a central line, measure urinary output, warm fluids
Activate massive haemorrhage protocol
Contact key personnel: senior anaesthetist, blood bank, haematologist
Arrest bleeding: surgical or radiological
Request laboratory investigations
Request suitable red cells
Consider cell salvage in appropriate situations
Request other blood products; platelets, FFP, cryoprecipitate
Consider drugs that decrease blood loss: antifibrinolytics, Rec Factor VII
Suspect DIC (disseminated intravascular coagulation)

What problems are associated with blood transfusion?
The transfusion of blood carries significant risks and problems.
The problems can be immediate or delayed.

Problem	Immediate	Delayed
Immunological	Immediate haemolysis, eg ABO incompatibility Graft-versus-host disease in immunosuppressed Febrile reactions	Delayed haemolysis: days 7–10 Rhesus incompatibility later leading to haemolytic disease of the newborn
Infective	Hepatitis, HIV, HTLV1, malaria, syphilis, CMV, glandular fever, brucellosis, vCJD, bacterial contamination	
Metabolic	Hypocalcaemia Hyperkalaemia: K^+ leaks in stored blood Acidosis Hypothermia Oxygen delivery is therefore affected by the leftward shift in the oxyhaemoglobin dissociation curve.	

Problem	Immediate	Delayed
Circulatory	Overload especially in the elderly Air embolism	Iron overload (chronic)
Respiratory	Acute lung injury/acute respiratory distress syndrome due to micro-emboli	
Clotting	Impaired by dilution and/or consumption of clotting factors and platelets Disseminated intravascular coagulation	

3

You are the SHO on call in a busy District General Hospital. You are asked to anaesthetise an 8-year-old child for manipulation under anaesthetic (MUA) + K wire of radius.

What are the main issues in your preoperative assessment?

Preoperative visit
Meeting with child and parents, history of presenting condition, previous medical history, previous anaesthesia, normal milestones/immunisations, family history, drug history, allergies, starvation time, weight in kg, EMLA/Ametop

Examination
Heart murmurs, breathing difficulties, activity levels

Investigations
Sickle cell

Current condition
Any cough/cold/temperature

Assessment of anxiety levels
It may be that premedication is necessary
Explanation what will happen to child and parent

Consent for suppositories

What should you have a high index of suspicion for in any child with a fracture?
Non-accidental injury.

If the weight of the child was not available how could you approximate the weight?
(Age + 4) × 2
(8+4) × 2= 24 kg.

How will you anaesthetise this child?
I would aim for an IV induction (with propofol and fentanyl/alfentanil) in this age group, but I would also contemplate a gas induction (with sevoflurane) if it seemed more appropriate or was requested.

If starved and the trauma was not recent, I would use an LMA. However, if I had any concerns over the stomach emptying I would use an ETT.

The weight is 24 kg so I would use a Mapleson E (Ayre's T-piece) or F (Jackson Rees Modification) circuit for induction and if available a paedi-atric circle in theatre. I would try to use scavenging on the circuits to minimise environmental pollution.

What size LMA and what size tube would you use?
I would use a size 2.5 LMA but have a size either side available if necessary.
I would use a size 6.5 uncuffed ETT and also have a size either side available.

How would you calculate how much fluid to give the child if you were just giving maintenance fluids?
I would use the 421 rule, 4 ml/kg per h for the first 10 kg (= 40 ml), plus 2 ml/kg per h for the next 10 kg (= 20 ml), plus 1 ml/kg per h for each kg thereafter (= 4 ml).

TOTAL = 64 ml/h.

During the procedure you notice the carbon dioxide is rising rapidly and the child is tachycardic.

What do you do?

This is a **medical emergency** and could be malignant hyperthermia. I would:

  Call for help including seniors, give 100% oxygen, hyperventilate the patient

  Prepare dantrolene at a dose of 1–10 mg/kg

  Stop volatiles, institute another anaesthetic, eg propofol infusion

  Change anaesthetic machine, tubing and soda lime

  Start active cooling

  Abandon surgery if feasible

  Discuss with ITU/PICU – correct DIC, acidosis, hyperkalaemia, promote diuresis

  Send clotting, ABGs, K^+, urine myoglobin, CK

  Treat arrhythmias.

Investigations

Serum CK elevation and myoglobinuria are suggestive but not diagnostic.

Follow-up care

Explanation to family plus follow-up of other family members

Refer to malignant hyperthermia centre where they will do caffeine and halothane contracture tests.

What are the triggers for malignant hyperthermia?

Volatile anaesthetic agents and suxamethonium.

What is the genetic explanation for malignant hyperthermia?

Autosomal-dominant inheritance thought to be on chromosome 19 or near to the gene for the ryanodine/dihydropyridine receptor complex at the T tubule/sarcoplasmic reticulum complex of striated muscle.

You are asked to anaesthetise an 87-year-old man for transurethral resection of the prostate (TURP).

What are the potential problems?

Related to the patient

Age

Neurological: mental state and communication, blind, deaf.

Respiratory: increased CV, decreased vital capacity, decreased chest wall compliance, decreased laryngeal reflexes.

Cardiovascular system: conducting system abnormalities, ↑ likelihood of ischaemic heart disease, ↓ cardiac output, ↑ circulation time, ↓ atrial pacemaker cell → atrial fibrillation, hypertension, ↓ catecholamine response. Uncontrolled heart failure carries a particularly high risk due to fluid absorption.

Renal: ↓ glomeruli, ↓ GFR, ↓ renal reserve, behavioural changes with incontinence.

Autonomic nervous system: ↓ ability to respond to stress, postural hypotension.

Skin: increased chance of peripheral nerve injury, less fat for warmth, thin/fragile skin.

Bone: decreased bone mass and strength.

Pharmacology: altered pharmacokinetics and dynamics. Reduced doses required.

Haematology: chronic anaemia.

Comorbidities: check for ischaemic heart disease, chronic obstructive pulmonary disease.

Related to the surgery/anaesthesia

Lithotomy position: pressure areas

GA vs regional anaesthesia:

GA. Disorientating, postoperative nausea and vomiting (PONV)

Regional. Difficult if patient is deaf. Obturator spasm → leg adduction. May need to decrease diathermy current.

Blood loss: preoperative haemoglobin, intraoperative loss is difficult to assess.

Use of irrigation fluid. Glycine may be absorbed → TURP syndrome.

Hypothermia: especially when large volumes of fluid infused.

Antibiotic prophylaxis.

Diuretic use: may request diuretic to flush bladder → hypovolaemia.

Postoperative pain.

Measure full blood count (FBC), urea and electrolytes (U&Es) the following day.

You opt for a spinal anaesthetic for the procedure.
What risks do you tell the patient about?
Technical failure and conversion to GA.
Headache: post-dural puncture headache (PDPH; 1 in 200).
Hypotension: common but treatable.
Pressure sores and chemical burns.
Rare but relevant direct nerve damage (1 in 10,000–30,000), spinal haematoma (1 in 150,000–300,000), spinal infection (1 in 150,000–200,000), total spinal.

What kind of spinal needle would you use and why?
I would use a pencil-point-type spinal needle that parts the fibres of the dura rather than cuts them and a higher gauge/smaller diameter needle (25 or 27 G), thereby reducing the incidence of PDPH.

What drugs would you give via the spinal route?
A local anaesthetic which is long acting enough to last the duration of surgery such as heavy bupivacaine 0.5% at a dose of 2 ml. An opioid can be given but is sometimes avoided in this age group as it can contribute to confusion.

Towards the end of the procedure the patient becomes agitated, restless and confused. What will you do?
Give 100% oxygen, call for help.
I would check the monitoring and the patient to see if there were signs of hypoxia, cyanosis, tachycardia, tachypnoea, or pyrexia to account for the acute confusional state. I would monitor GCS. If <8 consider intubation, check ABG, send bloods for FBC, U&Es, osmolality.
I would be concerned that the patient may be developing TURP syndrome.

What is TURP syndrome?
Fluid overload and hyponatraemia, which occurs with large volumes of irrigation fluid usually hypotonic glycine. The syndrome is also reported in other procedures involving irrigation such as hysteroscopic endometrial resection.
Syndrome consists of initially mental changes → visual changes → pulmonary oedema, cerebral oedema and coma.

How can TURP syndrome be avoided?

Patient factors

Ensuring the patient is not hypovolaemic or hypotensive as more fluid is absorbed in these states.

Blood loss; large blood loss implies a large number of veins are open.

Irrigating fluid – type and control of

Limiting the pressure of infusion: the fluid must be at 60–70 cm and not above 100 cm.

Limiting the volume of irrigant infused.

Monitoring of tracer substances, eg ethanol 10% added to irrigating fluid and monitored via breath or blood.

Anaesthetic factors

Signs will be detected earlier in an awake patient, eg spinal.

Avoidance of hypotonic fluids.

Surgical factors

Limiting the duration of surgery to <1 h.

Experienced surgeon.

List of Critical Incidents and Anaesthetic Emergencies

For each example discuss the causes, how it would present and how you would manage the event.
Most critical incident management should begin with:
100% oxygen, call for help, ABC.

Addisonian crisis
Air/amniotic fluid embolus
Anaphylaxis
Angioneurotic oedema
Arrhythmias including SVT
Aspiration
Bradycardia
Bronchospasm
Capnography alert
Cardiac arrest and peri arrest
Cardiac tamponade
Cyanosis
Disseminated intravascular coagulation
Eclampsia
Hypertensive crisis
Hypotension
Intra-arterial thiopentone
Intubation difficulty
Irreversible anaesthesia
LA toxicity
Laryngospasm
Malignant hyperthermia
Masseter spasm
Massive blood loss and transfusion
Oximetry alert and desaturation
Phaeochromocytoma
Pneumothorax
Prolonged anaesthesia
Pulmonary oedema
Septic shock

List of Critical Incidents and Anaesthetic Emergencies

Suxamethonium apnoea
Thyroid crisis
Total spinal
Ventilation difficulty
Vomiting on induction

Recommended Reading and Resources

There are many excellent textbooks on the market. There are some old classics which every candidate should read, eg West's *Respiratory Physiology* and other books which are an invaluable source of reference when facts need clarification, eg *A to Z of Anaesthesia*.

It can be useful to read the same topic in different books as it can improve your understanding of the subject. The internet is also a vast resource with a number of websites providing information and demonstration on topics relevant to the exam.

ANATOMY

Ellis H, Feldman S and Harrop-Griffiths A W. *Anatomy for Anaesthetists*, 8th edn. London: Blackwell Science Ltd, 2003.

Fischer H B J, Pinnock C A and Jones R. *Peripheral Nerve Blockade*. London: Greenwich Medical Media, 2004.

New York School of Regional Anaesthesia website http://www.nysora.com/.

PHYSIOLOGY

Ganong W F. *Review of Medical Physiology* (Lange Basic Science), 22nd revised edn. New York: McGraw-Hill, 2005.

Hampton J R. *The ECG Made Easy*, 6th revised edn. London: Churchill Livingstone, 2003.

Lote C J. *Principles of Renal Physiology*, 4th revised edn. Dordrecht: Kluwer Academic Publishers, 2000.

Power I and Kam P. *Principles of Physiology for the Anaesthetist*. London: Hodder, 2000.

West J B. *Respiratory Physiology: The Essentials*, 7th revised edn. New York: Lippincott, Williams and Wilkins, 2004.

PHYSICS AND EQUIPMENT

Al-Shaikh B and Stacey S. *Essentials of Anaesthetic Equipment*, 3rd revised edn. London: Churchill Livingstone, 2007.

Parbrook G D, Davis P D and Parbrook E O. *Basic Physics and Measurement in Anaesthesia*, 4th edn. London: Butterworth Heinemann, 1992.

PHARMACOLOGY

Calvey T N and Williams N E. *Principles and Practices of Pharmacology for Anaesthetists*, 4th revised edn. Oxford: Blackwell Science Ltd, 2001.

Peck T, Hill S and Williams M. *Pharmacology for Anaesthesia and Intensive Care*, 2nd revised edn. Cambridge: Cambridge University Press.

Sasada M and Smith S. *Drugs in Anaesthesia and Intensive Care* (Oxford Medical Publications), 3rd revised edn. Oxford: Oxford University Press, 2003.

GENERAL REFERENCE

Aitkenhead A R and Jones R M. *Clinical Anaesthesia*. London: Churchill Livingstone, 1996.

Hinds C J and Watson J D. *Intensive Care*, 3rd revised edn. Philadelphia: Saunders, 2007.

Pinnock C A, Lin T and Smith T. *Fundamentals of Anaesthesia*, 2nd revised edn: Cambridge: Cambridge University Press, 2002.

Yentis S M, Hirsch N P and Smith G P. *A–Z of Anaesthesia*, 3rd revised edn. London: Butterworth Heinemann, 2003.

OTHER RESOURCES

AAGBI guidelines. http://www.aagbi.org/guidelines.html
These guidelines are a rich source of up-to-date information and are likely to be used by examiners when preparing the exam.

Continuing Education in Anaesthesia, Critical Care and Pain provides monthly reviews on topics relevant to the anaesthetist in a supplement which comes with the *BJA*. There are also some practice MCQ questions after each article. **http://ceaccp.oxfordjournals.org/**

350

http://www.frca.co.uk/ has a number of practice exam questions and has a useful list of exam courses in the UK.

http://www.das.uk.com/guidelines/guidelineshome.html_ has algorithms for the management of difficult laryngoscopy, intubation and ventilation.

http://www.resus.org.uk/ has the latest algorithms for resuscitation.

http://www.mhra.gov.uk for information on adverse drug reactions, management of poisoning.

INDEX

Each locator consists of the question type, paper number and question number. For example:

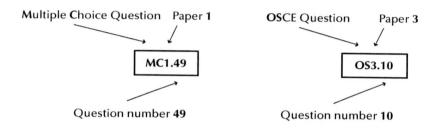

Multiple Choice Question   Paper **1**

MC1.49

Question number **49**

OSCE Question   Paper **3**

OS3.10

Question number **10**

Sphys1-10 refer to the Structured Objective Examination physiology questions, *Spharm1-10* to the pharmacology questions, *Spcm1-10* to the physics and clinical measurement questions and *Sclin1-4* to the clinical questions.

Notes

PasTest books in the FRCA range

Access to Anaesthetics: Primary FRCA Book 1 – Pharmacology and Clinical MCQs
Kirsty MacLennan

ISBN: 1 905635 29 X
978 1 905635 29 0

Access to Anaesthetics: Primary FRCA Book 2 – Physics, Clinical Measurement and Equipment MCQs
Kirsty MacLennan

ISBN: 1 905635 30 3
978 1 905635 30 6

Access to Anaesthetics: Primary FRCA Book 3 – Physiology and Anatomy MCQs
Kirsty MacLennan

ISBN: 1 905635 31 1
978 1 905635 31 3

"These books will give candidates a great chance of passing the FRCA. I can thoroughly recommend this Access to Anaesthetics series of books to all those planning for success at the earliest opportunity."
Dr David Whitaker FRCA, Hon FCARCSI, Consultant Anaesthetist, Manchester Royal Infirmary

Total Revision for the Final FRCA, Second Edition
Sarah Chieveley-Williams, James Holding and Tim Isitt
Reflecting the syllabus, this book provides MCQs, SAQs and VIVA practice papers that will prepare you for the entire Final FRCA examination.

ISBN: 1 904627 93 5
978 1 904627 93 7

How to order:

www.pastest.co.uk
To order books safely and securely online, shop at our website

Telephone: +44 (0)1565 752 000
For priority mail order and have your credit card to hand when you call

Delivery to your door
With a busy lifestyle, nobody enjoys walking to the shops for something that may or may not be in stock. Let us take the hassle out by delivering direct to your door. We will dispatch your book within 24 hours of receiving your order.

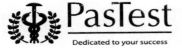